TOXIC INFERTILITY

Detoxification Solutions to Improve Natural Fertility

DEIDRE BLOOMQUIST

THE
SELF
PUBLISHING
AGENCY

Deidre Bloomquist
Toxic Infertility: Detoxification Solutions to Improve Natural Fertility

First Edition

Softcover ISBN 978-1-954233-32-4

Book Cover Illustration | Deidre Bloomquist
Book Cover Design | Tracy Hetherington
Book Interior Design | Petya Tsankova
Editor | Kathie Lynas
Publishing Management | TSPA The Self Publishing Agency, Inc.

Advanced Praise for Toxic Infertility

"The statistics around declining fertility rates are truly alarming - but there is hope. In her meticulously researched and highly accessible new book, *Toxic Infertility,* Deidre Bloomquist provides couples looking to conceive with a comprehensive roadmap filled with practical, actionable advice to boost fertility naturally. Bloomquist leaves no stone unturned, examining the many environmental toxins and lifestyle factors that can impair reproductive health. But more importantly, she equips readers with doable solutions to dramatically increase their chances of conceiving, maintaining a healthy pregnancy, and delivering a thriving baby. With infertility on the rise, *Toxic Infertility* is a must-read for anyone struggling to start or grow their family. Bloomquist translates the latest science into simple steps that can make all the difference in your journey to parenthood. I highly recommend this book to anyone considering conception! "

Margaret Floyd Barry, FNTP MRWP
Author of *Eat Naked and The Naked Foods Cookbook*

"*Toxic Infertility* has come at a pivotal time in our evolution. In my clinical and mentoring work, I've seen more miscarriages since 2020 than I did in the previous two decades of serving the birthing community. We need to start asking *Why*? As an active and "healthy" mama who miscarried 5 of my own 8 babies, I knew only to take nutritional support and had no reason to look at my toxin bucket. I didn't know to look and nobody made the suggestion, not even my trusted holistic practitioners. I missed the boat completely, suffered immensely, and it's likely you are as well. The mastermind behind this book, Deidre Bloomquist, shares her deep level of knowledge on why we must look at this and the steps you can take to support a more successful journey to fertility."

Nichole Hirsch Kuechle
Holistic Practitioner, Founder of My Healthy Beginning and Method of Intentional Inquiry

For every woman who feels like their body is broken
and that their day to step into motherhood may never come.

Table of Contents

The Beginning

In the summer of 2020, I found out I was pregnant with my son. We weren't planning to conceive at that time, and while I considered myself healthy, I hadn't had the opportunity to work on many of the things I would have liked prior to conceiving.

At that point, I had been a functional nutritionist for seven years and knew all about eating healthy, balancing meals, and using food as both nourishment and medicine. I had also been a full-time CrossFit trainer for years, and physical activity was something that had become a lifestyle for both me and my husband.

I had mercury amalgams (dental fillings) in my mouth, which, in retrospect, I would have had removed before getting pregnant. I hadn't had a chance to assess my microbiome and remove harmful pathogens or address lifelong, lingering digestive nuisances. I didn't check myself for mold and mycotoxins or prepare for pregnancy by reducing all environmental toxins throughout our home.

I had a wonderful pregnancy with very few symptoms and gave birth to my son, Jasper, at home. He was breastfed (and still is), and I was very confident about his health.

But when he was around six months old, I started to notice a dry patch of skin on his chest. Like most first-time moms, I consulted others. We sought out a naturopath for a second opinion, who said it was nothing to worry about. Over the next few months, a red, inflamed rash began to spread across his abdomen and onto his arms and legs.

When I realized I wasn't going to get the help I was looking for from other providers, I took matters into my own hands to assess my son's gut health, screen him for toxicity, and ultimately heal his gut. While that is a story for another book, what I learned is that I passed on most of my toxicity to him during pregnancy and was likely still passing toxins through breastfeeding.

I wish I would have been able to reduce my toxicity prior to him joining us in the world, to not only save him all of that pain, but also spare our family from the burden of feeling desperate and helpless. We were left stranded by conventional practices with no answers, no explanation, and no long-term support. It's a feeling I wouldn't wish on anyone as they grapple with the state of their health for themselves and their loved ones.

As a functional nutritionist, I've helped hundreds of women conceive when they've previously been left abandoned by conventional methods for supporting their health. Much like Jasper, I see these women struggle with surmounting toxin burdens and bodies that are crying out for help.

If you've been told "we don't know what's wrong or how to fix it," you aren't alone.

If you've been told that your chances of conceiving naturally are slim to none, and the odds with artificial support aren't much better, you're not the only one who has experienced that heartbreak.

If you've heard that there's nothing you can do to improve your fertility, you've been lied to – and it stops here.

While I was blessed to not struggle to conceive, I see how the same issues that plagued our family burden many women during their conception journey, and I've become passionate about ensuring women dig deep into their gut health and toxin status prior to conceiving – not only to help women who are struggling to conceive or carry to full term, but to also ensure their children live healthy and full lives free of the despair I felt through Jasper's eczema journey.

—

Stacy* came to us when she was 35 years old and experiencing a number of health issues that she was concerned about. She and her husband had discontinued the use of birth control eight months prior to starting their efforts to conceive but hadn't had any luck getting a positive pregnancy test up to this point.

**Name changed to protect privacy.*

When we met, she was experiencing very light periods that were lasting only a couple of days. She thought this might be due to coming off birth control in the recent past, but she had no idea how to fix it. She was also noticing hair loss and painful intercourse. When Stacy had contacted her OB-GYN about her concerns, they ran some bloodwork to make sure that she wasn't going into pre-menopause and also ordered an ultrasound to check for ovarian cysts. All of the tests came back normal, and ultimately, her OB-GYN suspected that she might have endometriosis. Like many women her age, she was starting to get concerned that pregnancy was not in her future.

At that point, they also tested her TSH (thyroid-stimulating hormone) and it was within normal range, but Stacy had noticed it was steadily creeping higher and higher. She felt like something was wrong with her thyroid but was still told "everything looks normal." She was feeling desperate as she worried she was running out of time to have the baby she had dreamed of and wasn't getting anywhere with her provider.

There was much more to Stacy's story before she went off birth control in her hope of conceiving. She also had a rocky digestive history that her OB-GYN had not asked about and wasn't considering as part of the big picture for her struggle to conceive.

A couple years earlier, she had developed a sinus infection and was treated with an antibiotic. Shortly after finishing the course of antibiotics, she was diagnosed with Clostridioides difficile (C. difficile), a bacterial infection that can be induced by antibiotic use. The C. difficile was treated and resolved in about three weeks, but for the next year she was extremely sick. She lost over 10 pounds and could eat only bland foods without experiencing stomach upset.

She decided it was time to see a gastrointestinal (GI) doctor and was prescribed proton-pump inhibitors (PPIs) to help her with the nausea she was experiencing. Her GI specialist recommended that she have an endoscopy, colonoscopy, and gastric emptying scan. She did each of these and was diagnosed with gastroparesis. Gastroparesis, also called delayed gastric emptying, is a disorder that slows or stops the movement of food from your stomach to your small intestine, even though there is no blockage in the stomach or intestines. Symptoms of this condition commonly include nausea, acid reflux, vomiting, abdominal pain and bloating, and changes in absorption, all of which can result in weight changes. Stacy was put on another medication to help block the nausea that often accompanies this condition.

She was finally able to eat normally after being put on these two medications and felt like they were managing her symptoms well, but her acid reflux had been getting worse over the course of six months. It felt like every day was different with her stomach issues, and she wondered if she would ever be able to function without these medications in her life.

To make matters a bit more complicated, a few years prior to the beginning of her GI issues, she started having fainting episodes. The first time she fainted unexpectedly, she fell so hard on her face that she broke her jaw. She had three episodes in a matter of a year, all centered around meal times. Her OB-GYN had suggested that it could be due to heavy periods, so she was put on birth control, and she didn't have any episodes for nearly five years until they picked up again. While she initially thought it had something to do with eating sugar and drinking alcohol, she experienced an episode when neither of those factors was at play, and she was stumped about what might be causing it.

One of the first things we noted was that her gastroparesis medication had an unintended side effect that might be inhibiting her ability to conceive. That medication was a dopamine receptor antagonist, which can increase prolactin production, while also suppressing the release of two hormones important for follicular development and ovulation: follicle-stimulating hormone (FSH) and luteinizing hormone (LH). We knew that helping Stacy ovulate and get pregnant might rely on helping her get off that medication, under the guidance of her prescribing physician. So that's where we started our journey, by getting to the root cause of her gastroparesis and upper GI dysfunction.

—

We have to stop thinking about infertility as a reproductive health issue only. While hormones can impair the ability to conceive, other systems in the body can create a state of stress that is a protective mechanism, signaling that it is unsafe for conception.

The whole-body approach to addressing infertility involves determining the root causes of infertility by addressing all body systems rather than just focusing solely on the reproductive system.

Many couples who can't become pregnant suffer from a combination of subclinical conditions. These types of conditions singularly don't cause infertility on their own, but in combination, they can substantially reduce a couple's probability of conceiving. Excess toxin burden and the resulting impaired digestion, gut infections, mold illness, liver toxicity, mitochondrial dysfunction, and hypothyroidism can all play a role in the inability to conceive. We'll discuss these concepts in depth throughout this book to help you determine which of these imbalances are creating stress on your body, as well as strategies to recreate balance.

—

As part of our initial testing with Stacy, we didn't conduct a single hormone test. Instead we ran a comprehensive stool analysis and blood panel. In her stool results, we found C. difficile still existing in the intestinal tract, as well as helicobacter pylori (H. pylori) in the stomach and multiple bacterial overgrowths. In her bloodwork, we found several indications of low stomach acid and insufficient protein intake, as well as subclinical hypothyroidism, despite her TSH being within normal range. There were signs of some liver dysfunction, and as one of the primary sites of thyroid hormone conversion, we knew that her liver needed some support in the aftermath of several medications and to ensure the organ could conduct its normal detoxification efforts for toxins it comes in contact with. We also found extreme immune dysfunction with low white blood cells and an immune system working hard against several pathogens. She also had low iron levels that indicated a mild anemia, likely as a result of her compromised digestion.

Despite the fact that she was taking a PPI to lower stomach acid levels and still frequently experiencing acid reflux, we were actually seeing that she had low stomach acid levels.

We worked with Stacy to soothe and heal the mucous membranes of the esophagus and stomach to first reduce her heartburn, and then remove it completely. This was the first step in allowing her to wean off of her PPI strategically, since it was no longer needed to mitigate her reflux. We also began addressing the presence of the H. Pylori bacterial overgrowth in the stomach that was contributing to many of her symptoms, including the reflux, heartburn, and inability to empty the stomach at appropriate times following a meal. By using herbal blends and upper GI soothing herbs, we were able to support healthy stomach-acid levels, and she was ultimately able to discontinue her gastroparesis medication without experiencing any symptoms.

We continued to address the downstream effects in the GI tract of this digestive dysfunction to rebalance the gut microbiome, replenish nutrient deficiencies, and ensure she was able to absorb and utilize the minerals needed to support thyroid function. We helped her to identify any sources of toxins in her home life that might be contributing to liver dysfunction and to support healthy stress levels through lifestyle changes and the use of adaptogenic herbs.

When we wrapped up our work together, we re-tested her stool analysis and blood panel. The pre-existing C. difficile was completely gone, the levels of H. Pylori had lowered significantly, and she had nearly rebalanced all potentially harmful bacteria to normal, healthy levels.

In her bloodwork, her thyroid that had previously been functionally depressed had come back into optimal range for the two main thyroid hormones, T3 and T4, and she was noticing new hair growth.

Her immune system had come a long way as well, with her total white blood cell (WBC) count coming back into optimal range. All of her immune markers returned to normal as well, indicating that not only had a huge immune burden been removed, but that her body was able to procure the nutrients it needed to mount a healthy immune response.

Lastly, her iron levels came back up to normal despite never supplementing with iron and instead focusing on her body's ability to chemically digest iron-containing foods.

A few months after re-testing, Stacy sent the following message:

"I just wanted to give you a life update. I found out this week that I am pregnant! Obviously it's very early. We weren't even really trying, and I honestly didn't think it would be possible before working with you. I wasn't even getting a period then."

This is what happens when we assess and address the body as a whole by focusing on imbalances, removing toxicity and immune burden, and allowing ourselves to heal naturally.

How to Use This Book

What you won't find in this book is a discussion of hormonal imbalances, different diagnoses, or how to track your cycle to conceive, and that's because your hormones are not the problem.

Imbalanced hormones are a side effect of a stressor on the body.

Your body is not broken. Your body makes no mistakes.

In many cases, the body is under such immense stress that it creates an unsafe environment for conception, and as such, we need to unravel those circumstances based on your unique situation, to allow you to heal.

The goal of this book is to help you understand the ways in which your body perceives stressors, both internally and externally, so that you can navigate the symptoms you're experiencing to dive deeper into your health. At its core, you must understand that toxicity is the root of all stress on the body. Toxins themselves dysregulate a number of systems in the body (including the digestive, liver, and endocrine systems), and as a result, create systemic dysfunction in various organs.

The symptoms we'll outline as we explore the contributing factors to stress on the body that impairs conception will help you understand areas you may need to dive deeper into, based on your unique situation. These symptoms are our body's way of communicating with us about the areas that require our attention and the areas under pressure. When we begin to unravel these symptoms, we can see how everything is interconnected and creating imbalances in the body that are perceived as an unsafe environment for conception.

When we remove stressors, we not only create an environment of safety for hormones to function optimally, but we can effectively reverse long-standing imbalances that result in common diagnoses such as polycystic ovary syndrome (PCOS), endometriosis, amenorrhea (missing periods), and even unexplained infertility.

Throughout this book, we'll help you understand the root cause of hormone imbalances and give you the tools to rebalance your hormones, naturally.

We'll first discuss the driving factor for all of these aforementioned imbalances, an unprecedented toxin burden in our daily lives, and we'll explain why this matters when it comes to hormone health and fertility. While you may have tried decreasing toxins in your personal care items in your venture to conceive a child, you may not realize how prevalent these issues are and all of the ways that you are exposed every day.

We'll then dive into changes you can make in your home to reduce your toxin burden and support your body's natural ability to detoxify. Addressing your environment is foundational to all other sections of this book, and it's paramount that you incorporate as many recommendations as possible into your life, even if done slowly over time. I can't stress enough that this step must not be overlooked. While you can certainly reduce the imbalances in the body that result from toxicity, if you do not address the causes of the toxicity in your life, you'll face these same issues again in the future. Creating a lifestyle that supports long-term detoxification will nourish your body for many years to come and establish foundational health for your children (and grandchildren).

While it can be overwhelming to understand all this information and the toxins we are exposed to through our food, water, and homes, it's best to consider implementing changes slowly over time. Perfection and zero toxin burden are not the goal. In fact, they are impossible to achieve. Instead, we want to lower toxin exposure as the root cause that leads to other areas of dysfunction throughout the body.

We'll then dive deep into a number of imbalances including symptoms you may notice in your own body and how to support yourself at home. In some cases, comprehensive testing is recommended. We always recommend that you test, not guess, when it comes to some scenarios, such as assessing imbalances of the intestinal tract's microorganism makeup, also known as its microbiome. Since symptoms associated with a variety of pathogens can present very similarly, it ensures your safety to properly assess and address the findings of testing.

In addition to testing recommendations for a variety of pathogens, we'll also provide information on affordable screening tests you can do at home and first steps to help support rebalancing, as well as things you can start implementing at home based on what you're experiencing. There are so many interventions that begin at home and drastically improve the quality of your life and your ultimate health outcomes.

The goal of this book isn't just to help you get pregnant. It's to help you get pregnant, have a healthy and easy pregnancy, support the birth experience you're hoping for by facilitating hormones not only now, but through the intimate workings of labor, and even support you into postpartum, with a healthy child free from the chronic disease so many children are plagued by. All because you decided to support your health now. You're doing powerful work.

Health is wealth, and your fertility is the most crucial component of exemplary health. I don't believe in gatekeeping the information that keeps many of us sick and infertile. We all deserve to have this information and guidance in our back pocket to incorporate into our lives and support ourselves. I hope this knowledge empowers you to take control of your health and that you will use it as much as possible to break the cycle of generational illness.

Why Doesn't My Doctor Know About This?

Medical providers have immense limitations placed on them, and unfortunately, they are in the business of "sick care." When running lab work, they are looking for markers to be conventionally elevated or depressed, indicating a disease is present. If most markers come back within their very wide conventional ranges, they simply see everything as "normal" and no cause for concern.

Physicians are also limited by their specialty and think of the body in terms of parts, rather than its whole. For example, an endocrinologist looks at hormone levels in the body without being able to look past that system, regardless of whether it's struggling or not, to ask what other body systems may be contributing to a decline in health. This means that if progesterone is low, rather than asking why that is happening, you may be prescribed progesterone to force levels higher in an attempt to conceive. Unfortunately, this approach does not account for the body as a whole. We are a sum of all our parts. The mainstream medical approach to health and fertility is to take a magnifying glass to just the sex hormones and organs, and ignore everything else in the body, even when it is screaming for help.

Physicians are also limited by insurance classifications, and while there are many wonderful doctors and I believe that all of their intentions are good, they are limited by their own education and the mindset to "fix an ill with a pill." As such, your physician may have never heard of the concepts or testing we will discuss here and finding a well-trained functional practitioner is something I recommend, whether you work with them in person or virtually.

DISCLAIMER: The content of this publication is for informational and education purposes only and is not intended to be a substitute for medical advice, diagnosis, or treatment. Please consult your physician for any medical advice. You should always work with a trained professional to analyze your symptoms, interpret the results of any functional testing, and establish a strategy for support in order to ensure efficacy and safety.

PART ONE

The Root Cause of Fertility Challenges

Chapter 1
A Challenge for Our Times: Declining Fertility

Infertility is a modern epidemic affecting more couples than ever. One out of six couples today experience difficulty getting pregnant, and males are thought to be solely responsible for about 20% and are contributing factors in another 30–40% of all infertility cases.[1] About 9% of men and about 11% of women of reproductive age in the United States have experienced fertility problems, with the issue being split equally among partners.[2] One-third of fertility issues lie with the male, one-third of issues lie with the female, and in one-third of cases, no cause in either partner can be determined. Depending on your age, couples have only approximately a 30% probability of conception using well-timed, unprotected sex.

In 2019, common causes of female infertility were broken into the following categories by the *Journal of Human Reproductive Sciences*[3]:

- 32% ovulatory disorders
- 12% pelvic adhesions
- 22% tubal abnormalities
- 15% endometriosis
- 19% unexplained infertility

Figure 1.1

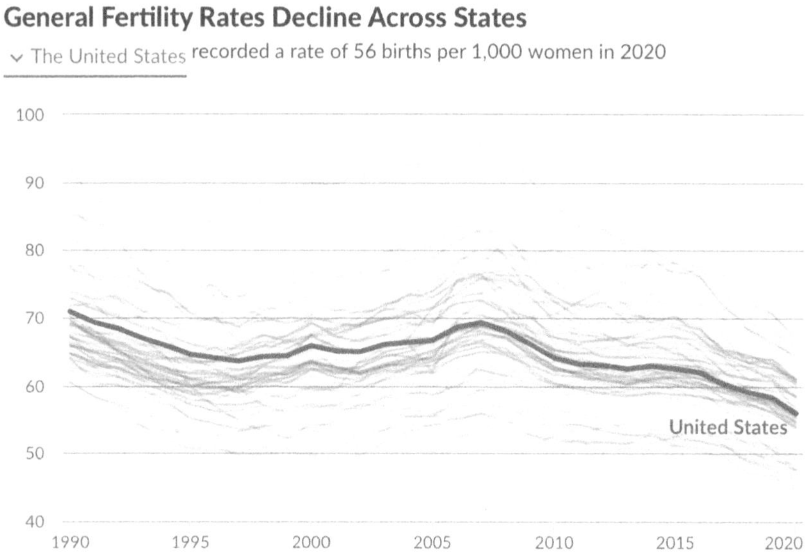

Source: Pew, 2022. The Long-Term Decline in Fertility - What It Means for State Budgets.

In her book *Count Down,* Dr. Shanna Swan outlines many of the factors contributing to an unprecedented decrease in fertility rates due to endocrine-disrupting factors, such as parabens, phthalates, and BPA, in our modern world. Swan predicts that by the year 2045, we will have a median sperm count of zero, based on following the curve from the 2017 sperm-decline meta-analysis.[4] This means that most couples may have to use assisted reproduction in order to conceive.

While infertility is a well-documented issue, causes of infertility for women surrounding the inability to ovulate are limited to the following, according to the Centers for Disease Control and Prevention (CDC):

- Polycystic ovary syndrome (PCOS)
- Diminished ovarian reserve (DOR)
- Functional hypothalamic amenorrhea (FHA)

- Primary ovarian insufficiency (POI)
- Improper hypothalamic or pituitary secretions
- Menopause

What these diagnoses don't help explain is why so many women are experiencing these types of hormonal imbalances during normal reproductive years. In fact, the only factors for infertility noted for women by the CDC are age, alcohol, smoking, being obese or underweight, and the physical or mental stressors that may result in amenorrhea.

Every day women come into my practice unable to conceive. Some have even gone through intrauterine insemination (IUI) or in-vitro fertilization (IVF) unsuccessfully, only to be told "we don't know why you can't get pregnant." The truth is that there are many factors within our control that put stress on our body from the inside, as well as external stressors.

Miscarriages

You've probably heard that one in four women will have a miscarriage. You might even be one of those women. And yet, if you've searched for answers about what causes miscarriage, you've likely come up empty-handed and are left wondering if you did something wrong or if there is simply something wrong with your body.

From 1990 to 2011, the risk of miscarriage increased by 1% per year among pregnant women in the United States, according to a 2018 study by the CDC. When we put this trend alongside the rising infertility rates and difficulties with conception, we have to wonder what factors are making it difficult to also sustain a pregnancy to full term.

Some miscarriages ultimately come with an explanation of chromosomal abnormalities, which is one of the leading factors in miscarriage. This means that the child was diagnosed with trisomy 13, 18, 21 (Down syndrome), monosomy (Turner's syndrome), or other sex chromosome issues. Chromosomal abnormalities may instead entail a molar (or partial molar) pregnancy, which occurs when two sets of chromosomes from the father are utilized in embryonic development.

But what causes these to happen? Is it truly a mystery that cannot be impacted in any way by our diet and lifestyles?

Aside from physical complexities, such as uterus abnormalities, some of the top contributing factors for the failure to carry to term in otherwise healthy women include blood sugar imbalances, infections, thyroid disease, low progesterone levels, excess oxidative stress, nutrient deficiencies, and mitochondrial dysfunction.[5] We'll explore all of these in detail, in addition to the driving factors for each, in the coming chapters.

Chapter 2
Surrounded by Unprecedented Toxicity

Our world has reached unprecedented toxicity levels through all of the things we come in contact with on a daily basis. This has been perfectly exemplified by a study showing the presence of 287 chemicals in the umbilical cords of children born in 2010.[1] Of those detected chemicals, 180 of them cause cancer in humans or animals, 217 are toxic to the brain and nervous system, and 208 cause birth defects or abnormal development.

Worldwide, the number of chemicals in commerce is estimated to be between 100,000 and 150,000, but since the registration of chemicals happens differently all over the world, it's impossible to get an accurate count. Not all of these chemicals are bad or harmful. In fact, many of them have made our lives easier, better, safer, and in fact, longer, but many others have proven to cause harm.

The core federal legislation in the United States responsible for regulating chemicals – the *Toxic Substances Control Act* (TSCA) – was passed in 1976. The TSCA took an "innocent until proven guilty" approach, which meant that chemicals did not need to undergo testing prior to being released into the marketplace; therefore, the only way for the Environmental Protection Agency (EPA) to actually regulate a chemical was to prove it was harmful after the fact.

In the United States, there are approximately 86,000 chemicals registered for use in commerce.[2] This includes 62,000 chemicals that were grandfathered in when the TSCA was passed.[3] This means 62,000 chemicals were given a free pass and an automatic presumption of safety without any requirement to actually test to see if they were indeed safe.

According to a report from the U.S. Government Accountability Office (U.S. GAO), the EPA has used its authorities to require testing of fewer than 200 of the 62,000 chemicals in commerce when EPA began reviewing chemicals under the TSCA in 1979.[4] While many women are aware of the need to reduce toxicant exposure during pregnancy, many women are not considering the cumulative impacts of exposure to toxicants over the course of their lives, some of which may still be residing in their body when the desire to conceive arrives. They're also unaware of how this toxic burden impacts other systems in the body outside of the endocrine system and how it can further exacerbate hormone imbalances as the body attempts to re-establish homeostasis.

Defining toxicants

"Toxicants" are any industrial or man-made chemical substances that impair normal physiological functions in the body, including hormonal, metabolic, and developmental functions. Heavy metals, such as lead, mercury, and arsenic, also fall into the category of toxicants.

The word "toxin" is defined as "an antigenic poison or venom of plant or animal origin, especially one produced by or derived from microorganisms and causing disease when present at low concentration in the body." In other words, toxin is a term reserved for substances that are produced by plants or animals.

I'll use these two terms interchangeably throughout this book, but it's important to understand that both toxicants and toxins have negative impacts on the body in similar ways. Whether we are producing the toxins within our own bodies, or coming into contact with toxins and toxicants in our lives, we all have a unique capacity for removing this unwanted debris from our sacred bodies.

We each have what I like to refer to as a "toxin bucket." When that bucket becomes full, it begins to overflow and this is where we start to see health issues arise. Think of a bucket that carries our toxin burden.

We all have a "hole" in the bottom of our bucket, physiological mechanisms such as bowel movements, sweating, respiration, and urine, that allow us to remove toxins from the body at different rates. Due to bio-individuality, some people are able to drain toxins through this hole so effectively, despite filling the bucket with toxins, that they never see the impacts of toxicity. Others have a very small hole to drain toxins from the bottom of the bucket, and as a result, their toxin bucket fills much more quickly. In rare cases, some people have no hole, or a clogged drain, which allows for these toxins to fill the bucket day after day without any relief until it eventually spills over. These are the folks who struggle with toxin burden quickly, experience chemical sensitivities, and see big health implications as a result of their inability to process the toxicity in their lives.

We all fill the bucket at different rates, based on what we eat and drink, the products we use in our homes and on our bodies, the air we breathe, the hobbies we hold, and so many other factors that we'll soon explore. Some of these factors are within our control, and some are not. While the goal is to reduce the amount of toxins and toxicants we come into contact with, the goal is also to reduce how quickly we are filling our bucket rather than never adding anything to the bucket.

While naturally occurring toxins are something that we have evolved alongside, and we have developed natural detoxification systems to remove them from our bodies, we're now being exposed to more toxicants than ever, which overburdens our ability to detoxify effectively. This toxic burden is not only contributing to a burden on our bodies, which we'll cover in more depth, but is also creating imbalances in our gut microbiome, reducing overall endocrine function, impairing cellular function, and creating deficiencies that all lead to hormonal imbalances and fertility concerns.

Let's discuss some of the leading types of toxicants that contribute to hormonal concerns, the inability to conceive, and miscarriages.

Endocrine-disrupting chemicals

The National Institutes of Health (NIH) defines endocrine disruptors as "chemicals that may interfere with the body's endocrine system and produce adverse developmental, reproductive, neurological, and immune effects in both humans and wildlife."[5] They are chemicals that can masquerade as estrogens, androgens, thyroid hormones, and even hormones like leptin and ghrelin, our hunger and satiety hormones.

While traditional toxicology posits that "the dose makes the poison," in the case of endocrine disruptors, extremely small dosages can impact the delicate workings of hormones and receptor sites in the body that rely on very low doses to orchestrate complex hormonal functions in the body. Tiny amounts of hormones can lead to profound effects on fetal and adolescent development and normal adult health.

In the book *Our Stolen Future*, authors Pete Myers and Theo Colburn describe just how minuscule the amounts of hormones in the body are: "Hormones are exceptionally potent chemicals that operate at concentrations so low that they can be measured only by the most sensitive analytical methods. When considering hormones, such as one of the estradiols, the most potent estrogen, forget parts per million or parts per billion. The concentrations are typically parts per trillion, one thousand times lower than parts per billion."[6]

These tiny levels of chemical messengers travel through the bloodstream until they reach their target receptors. Each receptor is designed to only respond to a specific type of message, or hormone. The endocrine system functions like locks and keys.

There are a number of different ways that endocrine disruptors do their dirty work, but the three primary ones are:

- They can mimic or partly mimic naturally occurring hormones in the body like estrogens, androgens, and thyroid hormones, which can inappropriately turn on or activate hormone response.

- They can bind to a receptor and block natural hormones from binding. When this happens, the normal signal fails and the body doesn't respond as it should.
- Lastly, they can interfere or block the way natural hormones or their receptors are made or controlled, for example, by altering their metabolism in the liver.

It's now estimated that there are nearly 1,500 chemicals that have been identified as endocrine disruptors,[7] many of which are found in the consumer products we buy and use every day.

While we typically think of endocrine disruptors for their ability to impact sex hormones, many of them impact other endocrine glands, such as the thyroid, which then disrupt the delicate balance of all hormones in the body. Industrial and environmental toxins also act as endocrine disruptors in their ability to impact thyroid health by displacing iodine in the body. Fluoride, chloride, and bromide all do this and are commonly used in the development of industrial chemicals:

- Perfluorononanic acid (PFNA) – industrial toxin
- Perfluorooctanesulfonic acid (PFOS) – chemical used in cleaning products, paints, paper, and textiles
- Perfluorooctanoic (PFOA) – chemical in detergents, dyes, non-stick cookware, and water
- Polychlorinated biphenyl (PCBs) – banned but still in environmental form in electrical equipment, paints, plastic, and wall coverings

Reproductive toxins are a subcategory of endocrine disruptors and do just what it sounds like: they interfere with normal reproduction, including through suboptimal fertility, infertility and sterility, miscarriage, and birth defects. These toxins directly impact fertility, while others we discuss may have indirect impacts.

Any chemical that is an endocrine disruptor, or any chemical that is a developmental toxin, can also fall into the category of reproductive toxin, and can interfere with both hormones (which are the primary drivers of reproduction), as well as with fetal development in ways that can interfere with that's baby's fertility in adulthood.

For example, the perfluorinated chemicals (such as PFOS and PFAS) have been shown to lower semen quality and testicular volume, resulting in male fertility issues,[8] and have been linked to increased risk of miscarriage.[9] There are hundreds of chemicals that can be considered reproductive toxins, and many of them have other effects as well.

Neurotoxins

Neurotoxins are synthetic or naturally occurring substances (like lead and mercury or certain bacteria) that damage, destroy, or impair the functioning of the central and/or peripheral nervous system. It's important to remember that the brain, and more specifically, the hypothalamus and pituitary, are responsible for the orchestration of all endocrine organs in the body and their release of hormones in the correct amounts to facilitate ovulation and pregnancy. While neurotoxins can contribute to neurological disorders and symptoms, we also want to consider the impact of neurotoxins on the brain's ability to facilitate healthy hormonal levels as well as conception.

When it comes to environmental chemicals, unfortunately, many of them behave as neurotoxins, and exposure to these chemicals can cause widespread damage.

For instance, a 2012 paper published by the NIH compared IQ among children whose mothers had been exposed to neurotoxic pesticides while pregnant to those who had not, and children collectively lost 41 million IQ points due to exposure to lead, mercury, and organophosphate pesticides.[10]

In 2014, two leaders in children's environmental medicine, Philip Landrigan and Philippe Grandjean, wrote the following in a paper published in the *Lancet Neurology*: "Our very great concern is that children worldwide are being exposed to unrecognized toxic chemicals that are silently eroding intelligence, disrupting behaviors, truncating future achievements, and damaging societies..."[11]

They go on to say in this paper: "Developmental neurotoxicity causes brain damage that is too often untreatable and frequently permanent. The consequence of such brain damage is impaired CNS function that lasts a lifetime and might result in reduced intelligence, as expressed in terms of lost IQ points, or disruption in behavior." Considering exposure to these toxicants is crucial in the preconception phase for ensuring the health of future generations.

They identified 12 environmental toxins as neurotoxins: manganese, fluoride, chlorpyrifos (a pesticide), DDT, tetrachloroethylene (also known as PERC, the chemical used in dry cleaning), polybrominated diphenyl ethers (PBDE) (these are flame retardants), arsenic, lead, mercury, toluene, ethanol, and polychlorinated biphenyls.

Chapter 3
Industrial Chemicals & Plastics

As earlier explained, the only way that regulators can remove or restrict chemicals is to prove they are harmful after they are already in the marketplace. According to a report from the U.S. GAO, the "EPA has rarely banned, limited the production, or restricted the use of existing chemicals. Since the Congress enacted TSCA in 1976, EPA has issued regulations under the act to ban or limit the production or restrict the use of only five existing chemicals or chemical classes."[1]

The five substances to be restricted or banned by the EPA include:

- Asbestos
- Chlorofluorocarbons
- Dioxin
- Hexavalent chromium
- Polychlorinated biphenyls (PCBs)

Unfortunately, even these five substances have not been fully eliminated as exposure sources for the public. Hexavalent chromium is a widespread contaminant in drinking water,[2] asbestos-containing products are still on the market, including in clothing, car parts, and cement products,[3] and dioxins are commonly found as contaminants in consumer products.[4]

It's estimated that around 1% of chemicals in commerce have actually been tested for safety, and even those that are tested have assumed safety rather than proven safety given the total chemical burden we face in modern society. This makes them not only pervasive and difficult to avoid, but puts us in a position where we may not know the true impact of these chemicals on our health and our fertility for decades to come.

Phthalates

Phthalates aren't a single chemical, but rather a class of chemicals used to make plastics more durable. As a result, phthalates are often called "plasticizers" and are used in hundreds of products, including vinyl flooring, lubricating oils, and personal care items. In personal care products, the four types of phthalates primarily used are diethyl phthalate (DEP), dimethyl phthalate (DMP), di-n-butyl phthalate (DnBP), and di(2-ethylhexyl) phthalate (DEHP).

All four of these are low-molecular weight chemicals, making them easily absorbable through the skin.[5 6] The most commonly used phthalate in fragrances is diethyl phthalate or DEP.[7]

In personal care products, phthalates serve to make fragrances last longer. They act as a fixative, holding the scent for long periods of times, usually hours. If you think about all the advertisements you've seen for long-lasting fragrance in your laundry detergent, hair wash, or lotion, you can be sure they are full of phthalates. According to the American Chemistry Council, diethyl phthalate can make up as much as 50% of the "fragrance" ingredient.[8,9]

While a single product may contain up to 300 different fragrance ingredients, there are over 3,000 different chemicals manufacturers can choose from, and there are no regulations to prevent them from using some known to be irritants and carcinogenic. Companies are not required to tell you how they made the product smell the way it does or disclose the chemicals they've used to develop their unique scent, just that it has "fragrance."

Because phthalates are so ubiquitous, our exposure is quite significant. In data collected by the National Health and Nutrition Examination Survey (NHANES), test subjects showed levels of phthalates present in their bodies, but the population with the highest levels of exposure was women of child-bearing age and those who were pregnant, who the most sensitive group to the hormone-disrupting qualities of the chemicals.[10]

Elevated levels of phthalates in the body function as endocrine disruptors by suppressing thyroid function, which can lead to weight gain, constipation, fatigue, infertility, abnormal menstrual cycles, and depression, among other things.

Phthalates exposure is also linked to:

- Male reproductive issues[11,12]
- Estrogen dominance[13]
- Female reproductive issues[14]
- Blood sugar dysregulation and insulin resistance[15,16,17]
- Decreased testosterone production in men[18,19]

While they're incredibly common in our environment, the good news is that phthalates are not fat soluble, persistent or bioaccumulative. This means that they are metabolized in the body at a consistent rate, typically 1–2 days, and therefore don't stick around for long periods of time. The problem, however, is that exposure is constant, which can result in elevated levels and health impacts.

Parabens

Parabens are widely used in personal care products, with between 75–90% of personal care products containing parabens.

Like phthalates, parabens are a class of chemicals, rather than a single chemical. There are five primary parabens that are used in personal care products: methylparaben, ethylparaben, propylparaben, butylparaben, and isobutylparaben. These are used as preservatives to prevent the growth of bacteria and microbes. Due to their molecular weight, parabens can pass through the skin and enter the bloodstream with ease, exponentially increasing their toxicity.

In relation to fertility, exposures to parabens have been linked to:

- Disruption of the endocrine system[20 21 22]
- Reproductive toxicity[23]
- Breast cancer[24 25]

A study done in Japan found that paraben exposure shortened menstrual cycle length in university students.[26] The Journal of Applied Toxicology released a study in 2004 that showed parabens present in every single sample of tissue taken from breast tumors, indicating a direct connection to the development of breast cancer.[27]

Plastics

Plastics are an inevitable part of the toxicants that we come in contact with on a daily basis. While we'll discuss ways to reduce exposure sources in Chapter 9, it can be helpful to understand why making a conscious decision to reduce plastic use is important for your fertility goals.

You've likely heard of BPA (bisphenol A) and are at least aware that it's something you want to avoid, but it's only one of many types of plastic that are adding to our toxicant burden. BPA is linked to hormonal disturbances, weight gain, insulin resistance, and early-onset puberty, among a long list of other conditions.

While BPA is not used in all plastics, it is representative of other chemicals and how they migrate out from plastics into the foods and beverages in contact with them. The chemicals used in the creation of plastics are not tightly bound from a molecular standpoint, which means that they can easily migrate out of the materials into the surrounding area. They are in a constant state of falling off and slowly shedding into the environment, which is a common theme you'll notice as we discuss the problematic nature of various plastics.

Since BPA is used in so many of the rigid plastic containers that we use in the kitchen, and since BPA is a well-established endocrine-disrupting chemical, this is clearly a problem.

BPA was first synthesized back in 1891, and its estrogen-like properties were discovered in the 1930s. It's been used as a plastic since the 1950s and reigns as one of the highest-volume production chemicals worldwide, with more than 10 million pounds produced each year, as of 2011.

A study done in 2003–2004 showed that BPA was indicated in 93% of people tested in the United States.[28] Another study found that for children at least, 99% of that exposure came from food.[29]

This is problematic, as BPA has been heavily researched and has been associated with:

- Metabolic disorders like diabetes[30]
- Insulin resistance[31]
- Obesity[32]
- Breast cancer[33]
- Recurring miscarriage risk[34]
- Early-onset puberty[35]
- Reduced sperm count[36]
- Low birth weight[37]

Most of the research around BPA points to its endocrine-disrupting qualities and the long list of health issues associated with it through that mode of action. But new research has found that BPA can lead to inflammatory bowel disease, which is a catch- all phrase to include conditions like ulcerative colitis and Crohn's disease, where there is chronic inflammation of the digestive tract.[38]

A study done in 2010 discovered that BPA from cash register receipts is readily being absorbed into the body just by handling receipts. In the study that produced this finding, the authors wrote that "experiments with viable skin models unequivocally demonstrate that BPA is readily absorbed and metabolized by the skin. The trans-dermal route is expected to contribute substantially to BPA exposure in humans."[39]

Bisphenol-A or BPA, is one member of a family of chemicals called "bisphenols." When companies sought out replacement chemicals to appease their customer base by providing BPA-FREE plastics, they simply turned to some of the other chemicals in the bisphenol family – specifically Bisphenol S (BPS) and Bisphenol F (BPF). These are unfortunately not any safer and in some cases are worse-offending endocrine disruptors.

A 2015 study on BPA and BPS in the journal Endocrinology stated that "BPA-free plastic products are not necessarily safer than products containing BPA."[40] Another 2015 study published in the journal Environmental Health Perspectives concluded that "based on the current literature, BPS and BPF are as hormonally active as BPA, and they have endocrine-disrupting effects."[41]

One of the most commonly used plastics is best known by its textile name, polyester, and is also known as polyethylene terephthalate (PET). PET is used in plastic soda and water bottles, bottles for juice, peanut butter, and condiments, and in frozen food meal trays, as well as some household cleaner bottles.

PET has been considered one of the "safer" plastics for use, which is why it's so commonly utilized, but this type of plastic leaches endocrine-disrupting chemicals, particularly phthalates, into the contents it contains.

The plastics industry has emphasized the distinction between PET and phthalates. In a letter to Environmental Health Perspectives, a spokesperson for the American Plastics Council wrote, "Plastic beverage bottles sold in the United States are made from a type of plastic known as polyethylene terephthalate (PET). Although polyethylene terephthalate (the plastic) and phthalate (the additive) may have similar names, the substances are chemically dissimilar. PET is not considered an ortho-phthalate, nor does PET require the use of phthalates or other softening additives."[42]

While it's true that phthalates are not used as substrates or precursors in the manufacturing of PET, several reports suggest that phthalates may leach from PET bottles into the contents of the bottle.[43]

A 2011 study from the Journal of Steroid Biochemistry and Molecular Biology compared waters from the same spring bottled in plastic and bottled in glass and found that "estrogenic activity is three times higher in water from plastic bottles."[44]

There are a number of things that increase the rate at which chemicals can leach from plastics. One of the most prominent is temperature, particularly heat. When plastic water bottles are exposed to heat, either by sitting in the sun, in the back of unrefrigerated trucks transporting shelf-stable products across the country, or in your car, leaching of chemicals is increased.[45]

Research indicates that when PET plastics are exposed to high, but reasonable temperatures, such as 90 degrees F, phthalates and other chemicals can leach into the water.

In addition to the leaching of phthalates, antimony can also leach from PET plastics.[46] Antimony is a silvery-white metal that is found in the earth's crust, and antimony oxide is added to textiles and plastics to prevent them from catching fire. It is also used in paints, ceramics, and fireworks, and as enamels for plastics, metal, and glass.[47] Many of the health impacts from antimony are from far greater concentrations than those elicited by PET plastics, but this helps to illustrate the fact that these plastics are leached chemicals in the products that contain industrial chemicals.

High density polyethylene (HDPE) is a stronger, more rigid type of plastic than PET and is used for things like opaque milk jugs, detergent bottles, bleach jugs, bottle caps, some types of food-storage containers, and thicker plastic shopping bags. It's relatively stable, warranting less chemical migration, but it can also contribute to endocrine disruption. Some research shows that an endocrine-disrupting chemical called nonylphenol, which is used as a plasticizer and an antioxidant in these polyethylene plastics, migrates out of HDPE bottles, including into milk.[48]

Polyvinyl chloride (PVC) is one of the most toxic plastics we utilize, and its toxicity exists throughout the manufacturing process and its intended usage. Its nickname is "the poison plastic."

While PVC is used in thousands of different types of products, such as water pipes, shower curtains, children's lunchboxes, and faux leather, in the kitchen, you're most likely to encounter it in softer plastics like cling wrap, plastic squeeze bottles, and cooking oil bottles. PVC is typically a rigid plastic. (Think about PVC pipes used in plumbing). In order to make it soft and flexible, various chemicals are added, including phthalates, lead, cadmium, and tin.

Even at the end of its lifecycle, when PVC-containing products are recycled, dioxins, one of the most potent carcinogens known to man, are a byproduct of the manufacture and burning of products that contain chlorine, including polyvinyl chloride.[49]

PFAS

Often referred to as Teflon, all non-stick cookware is made with a class of chemicals called perfluoroalkyl substances (PFAS), also known as perfluorinated chemicals or PFCs. The most famous chemicals in this class are PFOA, or perfluorooctanoic acid, and PFOS, or perfluorooctanesulfonic acid.

All the chemicals in the perfluorinated chemical family are designed to repel water and oil, and molecularly, they are some of the strongest bonds in chemistry. Because of the strength of these bonds, they are incredibly persistent in the environment and many scientists refer to them as being "virtually indestructible" or "forever chemicals." This means they don't easily break down, if at all, and they accumulate in the environment, as well as inside our bodies.

According to the CDC, 98% of the U.S. population has PFOA circulating in their bodies.[50] In fact, even polar bears and other animals in areas as remote as the Arctic have measurable levels of this man-made chemical in their bodies - and we know polar bears aren't using non-stick pans.[51] Because of its persistent and bioaccumulative nature, PFAS have a half-life that ranges from 3.5 years to 8.5 years,[52] which means that any given measurable amount will take 3–8 years to be reduced only by half, assuming there is no ongoing exposure.

According to Michigan State University biochemist Brad Upham, in a report published by the journal Environmental Science & Technology in 2001, "PFOS moves through the body by binding to blood proteins and subsequently accumulates in the liver and gallbladder. Scientists speculate that the body recognizes PFOS as a bile acid and continues to recycle it as it does with authentic bile acids. This recycling process, called enterohepatic circulation, begins when the liver uses cholesterol to make bile acids, which aid digestion by emulsifying fat in the gut. Once their work is through, the acids are recycled back into the liver."

This hepatic (liver) recycling is part of why this chemical appears in the majority of the population, as our bodies are unable to detox and excrete it properly.

Studies have linked PFAS exposure to:

- Reproductive toxicity
- Infertility in both men and women[53][54][55]

- Hormone disruption, specifically of estrogen and thyroid hormones[56 57]

A 2012 study of 10,000 children found those with the highest PFAS exposure levels were more likely to have thyroid disease – specifically hypothyroidism.[58] Because the thyroid affects nearly all body systems, any change in normal thyroid levels can lead to a cascade of negative health effects, including on fetal development, normal growth and brain development, metabolism, body temperature, muscle strength, appetite, and the overall health of the heart, brain, kidney, and reproductive system.

Prenatal exposures link PFAS to reproductive problems. Not only have studies in humans found a relationship between lower birth weights and concentrations of PFOA in umbilical cord blood,[59 60 61] but studies now show that PFAS are linked to miscarriage incidence. In a study conducted by the Danish National Birth Cohort between 1996 and 2002, researchers found that PFOA and PFAS were most consistently associated with miscarriage.[62] Miscarriage was also associated with the mixture of all seven PFAS being examined in this study.

Another study conducted by the Yale School of Medicine indicated a nearly 80% to 120% increased risk for miscarriage in women with the highest level of two common PFAS compounds, compared with those in the cohort with the lowest PFAS levels.[63]

Despite the fact that cookware companies reassure consumers that gasses only get released into the air at temperatures well above typical cooking temperatures, independent studies have shown that preheating a pan, as we often do, for only five minutes can produce temperatures where gasses will be released.

VOCs

Volatile organic compounds (VOCs) are chemicals that easily vaporize and are often inhaled in our homes in the form of household cleaners. While VOCs can contribute to acute symptoms (such as eye irritation, allergy attacks,[64] headaches,[65] nausea, fatigue, dizziness,[66] and irritability), they also have long-term impacts including:

- Decreased fertility in both men and women[67] [68] [69]
- Decreased testosterone levels[70]
- Decreased sperm counts[71]
- Low birth weight and other adverse birth outcomes[72] [73]
- Developmental disabilities and autism[74] [75]
- Miscarriage and increased rates of fetal malformations[76]

The main route of exposure to VOCs is through inhalation, which is one of the fastest ways for chemicals to enter the bloodstream. Under normal conditions, the toxicants we ingest have the benefit of undergoing detoxification in the liver, but in this case they are unable to directly enter the bloodstream via absorption through alveoli in the lungs. Furthermore, VOCs negatively impact the liver and kidneys, interfering with our ability to detoxify other toxicant exposures.

The household cleaning products that we use are such a significant contributor to air pollution that a study published in the journal Science in early 2018, conducted by researchers at the National Oceanic and Atmospheric Administration and the University of Colorado at Boulder, found that common household products like cleaners and perfumes rival the amount of VOCs produced by motor-vehicle emissions. They conclude that these everyday products are actually the top source of urban air pollution.[77]

Many household cleaning products contain synthetic fragrances, and with them, the phthalates known to impact fertility.

Glycol ethers are solvents used in degreasing products, with the most common type of glycol ether used in household cleaners being 2-butoxyenthanol. The types of products that often contain 2-butoxyethanol are glass cleaners, all-purpose cleaning sprays, and any cleaner intended for degreasing.

According to the Agency for Toxic Substances and Disease Registry, this chemical is linked to reduced fertility and low birth weight[78] and can cause birth defects in animals.[79]

Dioxins

Dioxins are released into the environment as a by-product of industrial activities. They're not actually created to be used for anything, but instead are simply an unintentional byproduct of incineration and fuel combustion. Dioxins are also formed, although to a much lesser degree, by things like forest fires or volcanos.

Dioxins travel through air and end up in water or on land, where they concentrate in our food supply. In fact, 90% of our dioxin exposure comes from food, much of that animal foods.[80] Seafood is definitely a primary source of exposure, due mostly to the fact that dioxins accumulate in fat tissues.

Dioxins, as is the case for PCBs, are linked to:

- Endocrine disruption[81,82]
- Reproductive problems[83]
- Breast cancer [84,85]
- Birth defects[86]
- Liver damage[87]
- Immune suppression[88]
- Fatigue and headaches[89]

Chapter 4
Heavy Metals

While heavy metal poisoning is the most commonly understood form of toxicity surrounding metals, heavy metal toxicity that is "subclinical" (not detectable by normal diagnostic tests) can include more subtle impacts to organ function and symptom manifestations.

Heavy metals are organic compounds that bind to parts of your cells, preventing your organs from doing their job. You'll notice that some heavy metals are considered neurotoxins, but their impacts reach farther than just impacting brain function.

While heavy metals can be contributing factors to infertility, difficulty conceiving, miscarriages, and birth defects, they also impact a number of other systems to create symptom manifestations, including:

- Neurological symptoms
  Cognitive decline,[1] memory loss,[2] ataxia,[3] tremors,[4] numbness and tingling,[5] neuropathy,[6] myopathy, Alzheimer's disease, multiple sclerosis,[7] paralysis,[8] Parkinson's disease,[9] tinnitus[10], irritability[11]
- Respiratory symptoms
  Lung disease, lung cancer, breathing problems, respiratory distress, pneumonia
- Cardiovascular and hematological symptoms
  Anemia, red blood cell (RBC) abnormalities, hypertension, low blood pressure, hypokalemia, edema, cancers of the blood
- Gastrointestinal symptoms
  Nausea, vomiting, diarrhea, abdominal pain, reduced absorption of nutrients (particularly minerals), dry mouth, metallic taste, pancreatic cancer

- Skeletal and bone-related symptoms
  Osteoporosis, reduced bone mineral density
- Dermatological symptoms
  Dermatitis, eczema, dry skin, sweating, skin lesions, hyperpigmentation, hair loss, allergic skin reactions
- Renal and liver symptoms
  Renal failure, elevated liver enzymes, hepatic damage, hepatic failure, suppressed hepatic detoxification, elevated hepatic enzymes

We all come into contact with heavy metals in some way, and while they impact us all to varying degrees, you may be more susceptible to the impacts of heavy metals if they build up and are unable to be detoxed appropriately, which is the case if you're exposed to high levels through drinking water, our food supply, beauty products, air quality, and vaccinations, or if you have poor detox capacity for genetic or other reasons. Orthodontic braces and retainers also release metals into the body. For those who have had long-standing orthodontic procedures as children, or still wear a retainer containing metal, toxicity from these procedures is worth considering.

Our ability to remove these toxicants effectively is what determines how much they impact our health. For example, MTHFR genetic mutations can inhibit the process of methylation in the liver, which we'll discuss in more detail in coming chapters. Methylation is critical for the removal of heavy metals from the body,[12] and with around 60% of the population having this genetic variation, it's safe to say that many of us are not supporting the biochemical processes needed to detox from the heavy metals we come in contact with daily. Heavy metal exposure can also contribute to the congestion of methylation detox, one of the crucial detox pathways in the liver, thus increasing serum homocysteine levels.[13]

Heavy metals bind to the sulfhydryl groups on proteins and enzymes in the body, and can then accumulate in the brain, liver, kidneys, and bones. This accumulation is a safety mechanism in the body to sequester heavy metals in specific organs and tissues to prevent the recirculation through the bloodstream of these toxicants. Recirculation on an ongoing basis contributes to oxidative stress and cellular damage. Think of oxidative stress as the typical trash produced through cellular function. Oxidative stress increases when cells are working hard to detox in addition to their typical cell function, and when antioxidants (the trash pick-up) is in low supply. It's for this reason that our body intuitively sequesters heavy metals. While this is not without health impacts, it's a safer option as our body does everything within its power to protect us.

Having a mineral deficiency (for example, low magnesium) also increases the risk for heavy metal accumulation, as the body will try to use the metals for the mineral enzymatic functions.[14] Therefore, any condition that depletes minerals in the body can create an environment that is more susceptible to the accumulation of heavy metals. This is often seen in secondary infertility or miscarriages following a successful pregnancy and birth.

According to the CDC, the "big four" toxic metals that you're most likely to be exposed to are arsenic, mercury, lead, and cadmium. We'll discuss each of these in depth, as well as two metals we see impact fertility, aluminum and nickel.

Arsenic is routinely detected in conventionally raised chickens and their eggs. It's routinely found in tap water, rice (particularly brown rice), seafood, and many pesticides. It is known to alter the lung-epithelial barrier (which protects and effectively clears the airways and lungs of inhaled pathogens and irritants) and to impede wound healing, as well as to be toxic to the immune system,[15] increase the potential for imbalances in the digestive tract, and cause intestinal barrier dysfunction (also known as "leaky gut").[16]

Mercury is one of the most insidious heavy metals with far-reaching impacts. In other words, it accumulates so gradually that its effects are not detected until it causes harm. One of the top exposure sources for mercury is in amalgam dental fillings, which can also contain cadmium, aluminum, tin, or copper.[17] Mercury vapors from amalgam fillings cross the blood-brain barrier and are known to affect hypothalamus-pituitary functioning, and therefore, the function of all endocrine glands.[18] We are also exposed to mercury from seafood, particularly large fish, and from the thimerosal used as an additive in annual influenza vaccines, among other pathways. In addition to direct impacts to hormone function, mercury is immune toxic and creates a greater potential for gut dysbiosis (imbalance in gut microorganisms), particularly the proliferation of yeast.

When you think of lead poisoning, you're likely to think of the severe impacts of lead toxicity, especially through gasoline and paint, where it was present until the 1980s. However, it still persists in the soil today. Other common exposure sources for lead include makeup, as lipsticks and mascara are often found to contain lead. High levels of lead can contribute to anemia,[19] weakness, and kidney and brain damage.[20] One of the key mechanisms of lead toxicity is the ability to damage and disable mitochondrial function, a principal regulator of essential cell processes including energy production. Furthermore, lead can cross the placental barrier and contribute to nervous system damage in children before they are born.[21]

We're primarily exposed to cadmium via the byproducts of smelting, the steel industry and waste incineration, through inhalation of polluted air, and consuming food and water contaminated with this metal.

Copper intrauterine devices (IUDs) can be a source of excess copper, as can hormone-replacement therapy and the birth control pill, as well as copper cookware and pipes. Copper is known to increase the likelihood of imbalances in the gut microbiome.[22] Copper is preferentially stored in the liver and the brain, and as a result, excess copper can increase the levels of estrogen in the body and prevent its detoxification.[23] At the same time, having excess estrogen levels and poor estrogen detoxification causes the body to hold onto copper.[24] This becomes a vicious cycle that contributes to hormonal imbalances, specifically estrogen dominance, whether it's excess estrogen production or excess estrogen relative to progesterone, and resulting in presentations such as premenstrual syndrome (PMS), breast tenderness, heavy menstrual cycles, endometriosis, and even estrogen-related cancers.

Nickel is very commonly used in a lot of medical devices, as well as jewelry, cosmetics, and cookware. Nickel disrupts the metabolism of hormones and lipids, and interferes with the production of the hypothalamic hormones and of luteinizing hormone (LH) and follicular stimulating hormone (FSH), which are responsible for the orchestration of ovulation.[25]

Aluminum is now being heavily studied in relation to breast cancers, specifically its role as a metalloestrogen (a metal affecting estrogen receptors.)[26] [27] [28] [29]

With all heavy metals, it's the longer, low-level exposure that causes the most harm.

All heavy metals impact the mitochondria's ability to function and produce energy,[30] which can not only impact systemic energy levels but also the ability to carry to full term.[31] In a study conducted in 2018, heavy metals were shown to cause miscarriages, even in levels lower than toxic doses.[32]

Arsenic, aluminum, and thallium in particular disrupt the enzymes that transport nutrients into the mitochondria in our cells.[33] Aluminum is also a neurotoxin and causes oxidative damage in the brain.[34]

Additionally, all metals have the capacity to induce what is known as a cell danger response (CDR) and impact immune system function.[35] Cell danger response is the evolutionary response that protects cells and hosts from harm, triggered by encounters with chemical, physical, or biological threats that exceed the cellular capacity to maintain homeostasis. CDR is one of the core consequences of a system overwhelmed by toxins. An immune system that is unable to function as a result of elevated toxin burden is one that is susceptible to all pathogens – bacterial, fungal, and parasitic.

Heavy metals can also mimic hormones,[36] over-activate or inhibit receptor sites,[37] and indirectly impact all endocrine function by disrupting hormone synthesis, displacing the minerals important for the function of these glands.[38]

All of the heavy metals to consider for toxicity and their impacts on fertility include:

- Aluminum
- Antimony
- Arsenic
- Barium
- Beryllium
- Bismuth
- Cadmium
- Cesium
- Lead
- Mercury
- Nickel
- Palladium
- Platinum
- Tellurium
- Thallium
- Thorium
- Tin
- Tungsten

It's important to understand that in an effort to protect itself from these toxic substances, the body will store heavy metals in certain tissues and organs to prevent recirculation and the damage that results from it. There are a number of ways to test for the presence and excretion of metals, but symptoms can tell you a lot about the toxicity of these substances as well.

While used as the conventional method for determining heavy metal poisoning, a targeted blood test can only indicate recent heavy metal exposure. More accurate testing for heavy metals can be done in one of two ways: urine or hair mineral testing. Hair tissue mineral testing shows long-term exposure to metals, as metals are excreted through the hair slowly while they may not be excreted via urine or blood, but testing of the hair is unable to indicate current exposures.

Urine testing shows current excretion and exposures, but can miss low levels of metals being stored throughout the body for self-protective purposes. If you have poor detoxification pathways, it's possible a urine test will show no excretion of heavy metals, even if you have confirmed metal in the body, such as in the case of amalgam fillings. Furthermore, urine testing results can be impacted by nutrient status, medications, calorie restriction, hydration status, exercise, and body temperature changes.

There is no perfect test when it comes to determining the presence of heavy metals, since they can be stored in several different tissues throughout the body, such as in the brain and bone, for which there is no way to test.

Chapter 5
Radioactive Substances

While the nuclear accidents at Fukushima, Chernobyl, and Three Mile Island may be relegated to the history books in your mind, we're still seeing their impacts on health now. Outside of the United States, there are 52 nuclear power plants operating without a license. Radioactive chemicals can also leak into the water supply from the Earth's crust due to processes like mining and drilling. The naturally occurring 1-trillion gallons of waste per year that oil and gas drilling produces most commonly contain Radium-226 and Radium-228.[1] While there is only one facility located in the United States dedicated to the permanent disposal of radioactive waste, the brine from drilling is often repurposed and sold as road de-icer and pool salts,[2] exposing the general public to these harmful elements in everyday life.

Think of radioactive chemicals like hot coals – they are always demanding energy from inside the body, pulling from the immune system and DNA to prevent damage. As a result, DNA is often damaged[3] by exposure to radiative chemicals, especially the DNA of mitochondria.[4]

These naturally occurring elements have toxic effects on the reproductive system, even decreasing conception rates. According to the Agency for Toxic Substances and Disease Registry (ATSDR), "If radium is swallowed in water or with food, most of it (about 80%) will promptly leave the bloodstream and be carried to all parts of the body, especially the bones. Some of this radium will then be excreted in the feces and urine on a daily basis,"[5] making healthy bowel elimination crucial. However, the half-life of these radiative elements depends on their structure. This is the amount of time it takes for just half of the radioactive substance to lose its toxicity. While Radium-223 has a half-life of 11.5 days and Radium-228 has a half-life of 5.75–6.7 years, Radium-226 has a half-life of 1,600 years.[6]

Uranium

Uranium is a naturally occurring radioactive material that is present to some degree in almost everything in the soil and rocks. While we all come into contact with some levels of uranium, higher levels can be harmful to your health. According to the EPA, studies conducted on the Navajo Nation among those who reside in abandoned uranium mines show an increase in autoimmunity, kidney disease, blood pressure, and impacted reproductive function.[7]

Uranium that is absorbed is deposited throughout the body, with the highest levels found in the bones, liver, and kidneys. Uranium's main target is the kidneys. Kidney damage has been seen in humans and animals after inhaling or ingesting uranium compounds. Ingesting water-soluble uranium compounds will result in kidney effects at lower doses. Uranium has also been shown to decrease fertility in some studies of rats and mice, even across generations.[8]

Uranium is a naturally occurring chemical element and part of the risk associated with it is the release of radioactivity. As such, uranium is a known carcinogen that was detected in 45 U.S. states between 2010 and 2015, according to the nonprofit organization, the Environmental Working Group (EWG). Uranium was found present at elevated levels in the tap water that serves 80-million people.

Figure 5.1

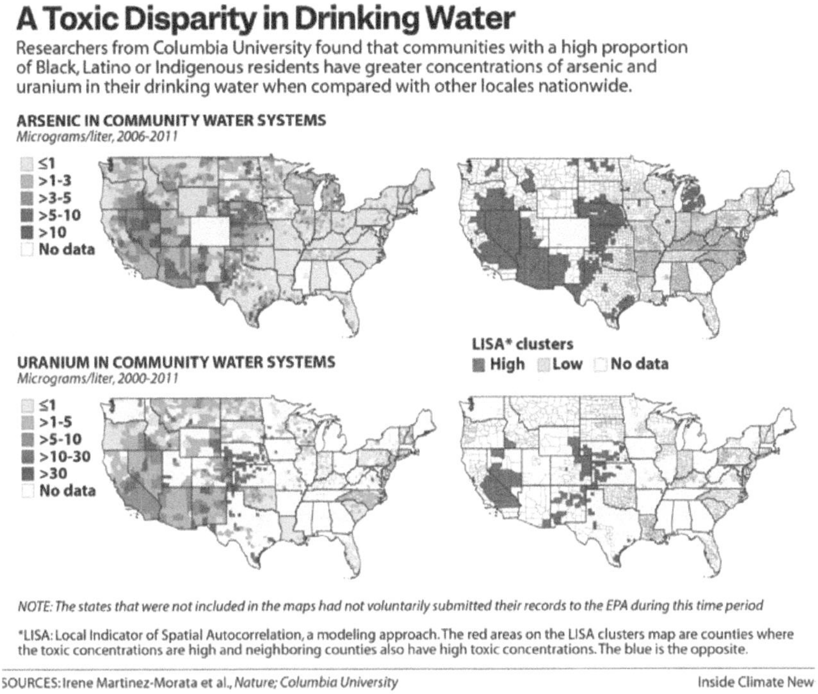

Source: Irina Martinez-Morata, et al. (2022) Nature, Columbia University.

Radium

Radiological contaminants like radium leach into water from natural deposits in the Earth's crust, as well as from industrial energy-extraction processes like mining, drilling, and fracking. Drinking water contaminated with radioactive substances is well-documented to increase the risk of cancer and may harm fetal development.

According to the EWG, 170-million Americans are drinking radium in their tap water.[9] If you're interested, you can visit their website (ewg.org) to see exactly where radium has been detected in the tap water, by ZIP code. Radium is 300 times stronger than uranium, and yet many people do not know they are consuming this daily in their drinking water.

The EWG collected data from public water systems around the country and analyzed five years of tests from 2010 to 2015. Radium was found in all 50 states, and they found 158 public water systems in 27 states "reported radium in amounts that exceeded the federal legal limit."[10]

According to that data, the state with the most widespread contamination is Texas, where more than 3,500 utilities serving more than 22-million people (about 80% of the state's population) reported finding radium present in their drinking water.[11]

Figure 5.1

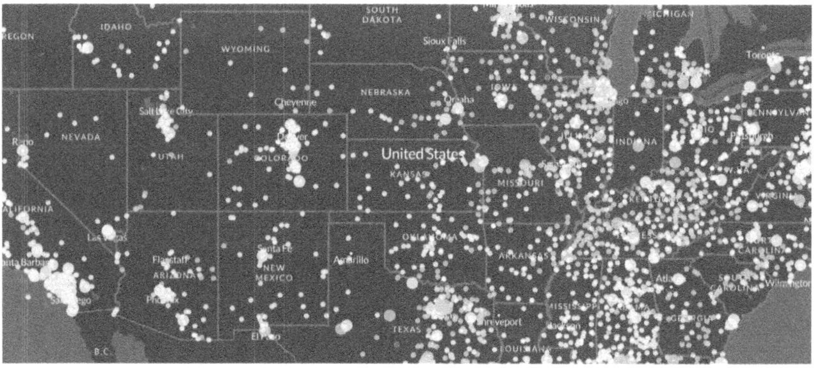

Source: Environmental Working Group. (2018). Radium Contamination in Public Water Nationwide

Symptoms associated with radioactive element toxicity include:

- Fatigue
- Anemia[12]
- Skin issues[13]
- Hair loss[14]
- Dry eyes[15]
- Seizures[16]
- History of cancer
- Chronic candida infections[17]
- Hormone or fertility problems[18][19]

- Suppression of immune function and autoimmunity[20]
- Osteoporosis
- Kidney or urinary problems (bladder infections, burning/pain with urination)[21]
- Digestive problems (difficulty swallowing, dry mouth, stomach ulcers, taste changes)

Most exposure of radioactive chemicals comes from drinking water. Radon in particular can be inhaled and impact the lungs, which is why in many states, radon detection is required when buying a home.

Chapter 6
Pesticides & Herbicides

Pesticides are something we don't typically consider in our daily lives or acknowledge are being used on virtually every produce item and crop produced, not only in the United States, but globally. For our purposes, pesticides will include herbicides (weed killers), fungicides (fungus killers), insecticides (insect killers), and rodenticides (rodent killers). These chemicals are used to prevent the infestation of these "pests" that damage crop yields and are also used in residential settings, including lawns, golf courses, forests, and farms.

You might be familiar with DDT (Dichlorodiphenyltrichloroethane) as one of the most harmful pesticides ever used in agriculture. It was the first modern synthetic pesticide classified as an organochloride and was used heavily during World War II to control the insects that were spreading typhus. It was later used to wipe out malaria in Europe and North America.

DDT was banned for use in the United States in 1972 due to its adverse environmental effects, including on wildlife, as well as its potential human health risks. Since its removal from use, studies have continued to show a relationship between DDT exposure and reproductive effects in humans.[1]

Like all organochloride pesticides, DDT is lipophilic and is stored in the fatty parts of our bodies, such as adipose (fat) tissue, the liver, and the brain. As a result, both blood and urine testing for these compounds are considered to produce results that underestimate the true body burden.

Even after being phased out in the 1970s, DDT and its metabolites have been measured in umbilical cord blood as recently as 2010,[2] and I frequently see DDT metabolites present in the urine of women struggling to conceive. It's also not uncommon to see DDT detected in people born after the '70s, due to the transfer of toxins from mothers to their children while in utero.

This is important to note because even low-dose exposures to DDT are associated with:

- Early onset puberty and shortened length of menstruation[3]
- Trouble conceiving in women[4]
- Fertility issues in men[5]
- Low birth weight, which on its own can lead to developmental issues[6]
- Poor attention in children born to mothers with low levels of DDT[7]
- Blood sugar dysregulation and diabetes[8]
- Autism[9]

According to the Agency for Toxic Substances and Disease Registry, the half-life of DDT depends on the soil type but varies from 2 to 15 years.[10] This means that while DDT is not currently being sprayed on crops, it may still exist in the soil and be contaminating not only crops being grown today, but also water sources.

Glyphosate

Following the ban on DDT in 1972, glyphosate was registered for use as a pesticide in 1974 and has been gaining momentum in use ever since. Before it was patented as a herbicide, glyphosate was first patented as a metal chelator in 1961 and was originally designed to clean mineral scaling out of boiler systems. This is an important component of its function that we'll return to.

Glyphosate is a widely used herbicide and the declared active ingredient in RoundUp®, which controls broadleaf weeds and grasses. It is the most widely used herbicide in the world and may very well go down in history as the DDT of our generation.

Before we dig into why it's so dangerous, let's discuss how its widespread use came to be. Following its introduction in 1974, its use has increased dramatically in the past 20 years due to the frequent use of crop seeds genetically modified to withstand the use of pesticides to increase output, also known as Roundup crops, including corn, soybean, cotton, and wheat, as well as fruits and vegetables. Approximately 3.42-billion pounds of glyphosate are applied annually worldwide,[11] with China being both the largest producer and user of glyphosate. It's worth noting here that China also produces most organic foods and is not as diligent as other countries about ensuring agricultural processes are respected for certified organic foods.[12]

According to the EPA, agricultural uses include corn, cotton, canola, soybean, sugar beet, alfalfa, berry crops, Brassica vegetables, bulb vegetables, fruiting vegetables, leafy vegetables, legume vegetables, cucurbit vegetables, root tuber vegetables, cereal grains, grain sorghum, citrus crops, fallow, herbs and spices, orchards, tropical and subtropical fruits, stone fruits, pome fruits, nuts, vine crops, oilseed crops, and sugarcane. Nonagricultural uses include conservation land, pastures, rangeland, aquatic areas, forests, turf grass, residential areas, non-food tree crops (e.g., pine, poplar, Christmas trees), rights of way, commercial areas, paved areas, spot treatments, ornamentals, parks, and wildlife management areas.[13]

As you can see, there are several routes for exposure that are dependent on where you live, what type of food you eat, and where you spend your time. An article published in the *Journal of the American Medical Association* (JAMA) found that the percentage of people who tested positive for glyphosate and its primary metabolite shot up 500% in the years between 1993 and 2016.[14]

The impacts of glyphosate are systemic and far-reaching, and exposure has been associated with:

- Increased risk of miscarriage and pre-term births[15]
- Oxidative damage
- Neurotoxicity[16]
- Breast cancer cell proliferation[17]
- Neurobehavioral disorders, including ADHD[18]

Scholars indicate that glyphosate is also a factor in the decreasing microbial diversity in soil that contributes to erosion, lack of nutrients in agricultural land, and the resulting changes to nutrient density in the food grown on land contaminated by glyphosate.

Impacts on digestion

Glyphosate disrupts the ability of the digestive enzymes of trypsin, pepsin, and lipase to digest food chemically. Intestinal paralysis is one of the severe reactions to acute glyphosate exposure, and chronic exposure can cause constipation.

Glyphosate also acts like an antibiotic that may alter the GI microbiome in ways that could favor the proliferation of pathogenic microbes. In fact, in 2010, glyphosate was patented as a broad-spectrum antibiotic. This means that it's not strain-specific as many antibiotics are, and that it causes widespread damage to bacteria of varying strains. It can also contribute to antibiotic resistance. This means that we can become infected with bacteria that are less likely to be eradicated with the use of antibiotics. A 2015 study found that environmentally relevant exposures to glyphosate altered the susceptibility of bacteria to six classes of antibiotics.[19] According to the CDC's 2019 Antibiotic Resistance Threats Report, more than 2.8-million antimicrobial-resistant infections, such as C. difficile, occur each year in the United States, with more than 35,000 people dying as a result.[20]

Glyphosate also contributes to overgrowths in harmful bacteria in the gut microbiome through antibiotic-like reactions that alter the microbiome as well. The Pseudomonas species of bacteria has been well studied with respect to its ability to metabolize glyphosate, resulting in overgrowths of this bacteria in the microbiome.[21] Glyphosate also significantly disrupts the function of beneficial bacteria in the microbiome and contributes to intestinal permeability, which we'll discuss more in Chapter 13. This suppression of beneficial bacteria also contributes to immune impairment as a whole.

Impacts on the liver

Glyphosate is specifically toxic to the liver, which is often the first organ impacted by glyphosate exposure. Glutathione is one of the key detox enzymes that helps our liver to metabolize toxins. Glutathione is depleted by glyphosate, which contributes to systemic oxidative stress, mitochondrial impairment, and DNA damage, and glyphosate is a leading factor in fatty liver disease.[22] Glyphosate also appears to directly alter our ability to detoxify other chemicals or substances like arsenic, by depleting levels of glutathione in the body.

One of the most profound impacts of glyphosate is the disruption of cytochrome P459 (CYP) enzymes, which detoxify a multitude of foreign chemicals and compounds, including xenobiotics.[23] Xenobiotics are synthetic substances and chemicals that account for 80–90% of chemical toxicity in the human population, which makes the detoxification of these substances crucial.[24]

Research on rats showed that glyphosate contributed to elevated levels of AST and ALT liver enzymes in blood serum, as well as elevated levels of urea and creatinine (metabolic waste products carried to the kidney), showing impacts to both the liver and kidneys by weakening their efficiency as crucial detoxification pathways.[25] Another study showed impacts on total cholesterol, LDL, and triglyceride elevations, which imply that glyphosate can be contributing to the epidemic of cardiovascular disease.[26]

As a heavy metal chelator, glyphosate can mobilize heavy metals throughout the body, removing them from safe sequestration in various tissues. This means that heavy metals can have a great impact on liver function, as well as the immune system, depending on the metal being mobilized.

Impacts on the immune system

Glyphosate alters the complement cascade of the immune system,[27] which is the process of antibodies binding to foreign particles for elimination, as well as the ability of phagocytes (a category of immune cells) to function in the ingestion of microbial pathogens.[28] Both of these systemic effects can increase the susceptibility of pathogens to overtake the immune system.

Glyphosate also increases the production of pro-inflammatory cytokines.[29] Cytokines are small proteins that immune cells release as part of cell signaling in response to the exposure to a variety of things in the body. For instance, cytokines can be released to create an inflammatory response in response to food antigens, which therefore creates an inflammatory response in the body. As such, cytokines are used to regulate inflammation in an attempt to heal tissues of the body, but this becomes problematic when inflammation is systemic.

Glyphosate can also contribute to autoimmunity. The chemical modification of food proteins by these toxicants may result in immune reactions against modified food proteins, which cross-react with tissue antigens, resulting in autoimmune reactivity.[30]

Impacts on hormones

Glyphosate is a known and well-documented endocrine disruptor and a leading factor in infertility, miscarriages, and premature births, as well as intrauterine growth restrictions and fetal malformations.[31] It mimics estrogen and has been correlated to aggressive breast cancers. All levels of the hypothalamic-pituitary-gonadal system that regulate fertility are impacted by exposure to glyphosate, including the ovaries, testes, uterus, and placenta.[32]

According to Stephanie Seneff, one of the leading researchers in the health impacts of glyphosate, "While the research literature on glyphosate's endocrine disrupting effects is limited, diverse evidence from animal studies reveals effects that suggest impaired thyroid function in both the mother and in the fetus."[33]

We'll discuss exposure sources, strategies from reducing exposure, and a plan of action for supporting detoxification, in more depth in Chapter 9.

While glyphosate is one of the biggest offenders among chemical sprays impacting our health, organophosphate (OP) pesticides are also worth considering in terms of their role in chemical toxicity. First, we need to understand how OP pesticides have been introduced and why it matters from a historical perspective.

Organochloride pesticides began being used in the 1930s, as insecticides. They are endocrine-disrupting, lipophilic substances that have very long half-lives, and they don't break down in the environment. Due to their persistent qualities and clear toxicity to humans and animals, they have been largely phased out of use.

Next came organophosphate pesticides, which were introduced as a safer alternative to organochlorides. Organophosphate pesticides are designed to interfere with the central nervous system of insects by inhibiting an enzyme called acetylcholinesterase. Acetylcholine is a neurotransmitter that plays an important role in the firing of our neurons. Too much acetylcholine can cause neurons to misfire, which results in sending mixed messages throughout the body, consistent with symptoms found in autistic people, those with mental disorders, and conditions like epilepsy. Normally, the body keeps excess acetylcholine in check through this acetylcholinesterase enzyme. Organophosphate pesticides inhibit this enzyme, which results in the nervous system becoming severely overstimulated and neurological dysfunction.[34]

While exposure to high doses of organophosphates can cause headaches, twitching, trembling, the inability to breathe via paralysis of the diaphragm, convulsions, and even death, low levels of exposure are linked to chronic fatigue,[35] reduced IQ in children,[36] neurobehavioral development issues,[37] ADHD,[38] and you guessed it – reproductive effects for both men and women.[39] In fact, exposure to these pesticides has been shown to alter levels of follicle-stimulating hormone production in the brain, which is responsible for facilitating the release and maturation of eggs for fertilization.[40]

Chlorpyrifos

Of note is one organophosphate pesticide – chlorpyrifos. This pesticide was banned for residential use more than 20 years ago, but is still widely used in the United States on more than 60 food crops, primarily in California. It remains one of the top pesticides used around the world on crops like corn, soybeans, wheat, cotton, and grapes and wine orchards, among others.[41] They're also used on bananas, apples, and even Christmas trees.

Newer research has shown that chronic, low-dose exposure to chlorpyrifos can induce dysbiosis in the microbial community of the gut in rodent studies.[42] In other words, it disrupts the balance of our gut bacteria.

Another study on chlorpyrifos found that it caused gut microbiome alterations that resulted in intestinal inflammation and abnormal intestinal permeability, otherwise popularly known as "leaky gut."[43]

Chlorpyrifos also significantly impacts the release of gonadotropin-releasing hormone in the hypothalamus, which plays an integral role in the orchestration of all endocrine glands.[44]

Atrazine

Atrazine is a chlorinated triazine systemic herbicide that is used to selectively control annual grasses and broadleaf weeds before they emerge. Several agricultural crops utilize atrazine, including field corn, sweet corn, sorghum, sugarcane, wheat, macadamia nuts, and guava. It is also used for non-agricultural purposes such as for nursery/ornamental plants and turf.

The European Union banned its use in 2004, but the EPA in the United States currently regulates atrazine to be limited to 3 ppb in drinking water. Atrazine (75 mg/kg) both activated the release of pituitary hormones and inhibited luteinizing hormone (LH) release from the pituitary in rats.[45]

Atrazine has been implicated as an endocrine-disrupting chemical that alters reproductive function by targeting the hypothalamic-pituitary-gonad axis. Male mammalian models have begun to be of key importance in understanding reproductive dysfunction, with gestational exposure demonstrating a delay in puberty.

Furthermore, prenatal and adult studies show decreased levels of testosterone and altered testicular morphology in response to atrazine exposure. Steroidogenic genes and upstream regulators are altered due to atrazine exposure, in both granulosa cells (in the ovaries) and Leydig cells (in the testes). Aquatic studies have observed decreases in spawning events and egg production, alterations in hormone levels and gonad histology, and genetic changes.[46] One of the most prominent studies conducted on atrazine involved African frogs, where exposure to the herbicide induced chemical castration and the complete feminization of male frogs.[47] Atrazine-exposed males suffered from depressed testosterone, decreased breeding gland size, demasculinized/feminized laryngeal development, suppressed mating behavior, reduced spermatogenesis, and decreased fertility, which is consistent with research conducted on other vertebrates.

It's clear that while our food choices are of utmost importance, what is being sprayed on our food, found in the soil in which it grows, and contaminating the water nourishing our produce, livestock, and us is equally as important in the consideration of total toxicity for the health of our hormones.

Chapter 7
Mold & Mycotoxins

Not all toxins are man-made, however. Nature produces its own form of toxins, known as biotoxins, that are equally as detrimental to our health. In our modern world, these biotoxins are becoming increasingly prevalent due to the limitation of nature forces that have kept their proliferation in check. For even the most seasoned of toxin-free lifestyles, mold is often missed, and the impacts to fertility and miscarriage are monumental.

The two most common mycotoxins we see impacting fertility are Ochratoxin A (OTA) and Zearalenone (ZEA). OTA can come from both environmental sources, such as water-damaged buildings, as well as poorly stored food products, and inhibits mitochondrial function as well as poisons the immune system and kidneys.

On the other hand, ZEA deserves special note. It is a non-steroidal estrogenic mycotoxin that contaminates grains such as maize, wheat, barley, oats, rye, sorghum, millet, and rice that we commonly see in women experiencing hormonal imbalances. ZEA and its metabolites bind the estrogen receptors sites, effectively acting as an endocrine disruptor and disrupting the feedback communication to the pituitary.[1] As a result, women often experience symptoms that resemble estrogen dominance, such as heavy periods, clotting, breast tenderness, and PMS, but upon further testing, their estrogen levels are actually low, as ZEA signals to the pituitary that adequate estrogen is being produced.[2] It has been documented to cause fertility issues,[3] the proliferation of estrogen-dependent cells, reproductive and breast cancers,[4] and pregnancy loss.[5]

It's easy to think about mold as an issue that only happens in unkept home and that when there's a mold problem, you can always see it. The truth is that mold exists in about 70% of homes in the United States,[6] and its presence isn't always obvious because mold can grow on a wide number of surfaces. Mold only requires two things to grow: humidity and darkness.

The number one source of exposure to mold, by far, is water-damaged buildings, as molds can grow on almost any wet and warm place, including inner walls of buildings, fiberglass insulation, and wallpaper, amongst others. According to the 2005 Federal Facilities Council's review, Implementing Health-Protective Features and Practices in Buildings, 43% of buildings examined had current water damage, and 85% had past water damage. With water damage, mold can begin to grow in as few as 48 hours, and 66% of materials from water-damaged buildings contain molds and their resulting toxins.

Mold isn't just an issue in old homes; new builds are often more susceptible to mold presence. Poor building methods also contribute, for example, airtight new homes, basements and crawl spaces, installation of moldy materials, such as wet framing wood, HVAC and plumbing errors, high indoor humidity and condensation, appliances, fish tanks, and plants. Poor upkeep can be the problem, especially in institutional buildings such as schools and hospitals.

It's important to understand that mold is not inherently dangerous, and it's a normal part of life – a presence that we have evolved alongside for centuries. Mold is not dangerous in nature because it can be kept in check via sun exposure and fresh air.

In our homes, where sunlight often does not reach, and in airtight homes, where fresh air rarely reaches (especially in certain climates), it's not uncommon to see worse air quality as well as high levels of mold and their resulting mycotoxins.

While mold is important to address from a current exposure standpoint, mycotoxins from mold are what impact our health.

Molds produce airborne spores, and some of these spores produce toxins called mycotoxins. Mycotoxins are poisonous substances produced mainly by fungi, including molds. These biotoxins are some of the most impactful and commonly missed stressors to the body that can impact the fertility of both men and women, due to their wide-reaching and complex effects.

These fungal overgrowths don't impact everyone in the same way, and poor detoxification, as well as impaired immune function, are some of the biggest factors that determine how severely they impact your health. If you're coming into contact with high levels of toxins, such as heavy metals, you become a susceptible host for mycotoxins.

According to Dr. Dietrich Klinghardt, "Toxic metals harm the cells of the body whereas the invading microbes (including mold) thrive in a heavy metal environment. Research by Ludwig, Voll, and others in Germany and by Omura and myself here in the US, show that microbes tend to set up their housekeeping in those body compartments that have the highest pollution with toxic metals."[7]

How do we come in contact with mycotoxins?

Mold spores, spore fragments, and mycotoxins are most commonly inhaled, but exposure can also occur by skin contact and consumption.

Over 1,000 different mycotoxins have been identified. They exist to provide competitive inhibition, killing off other microbes so that the mold can spread and thrive. Antibiotics, such as penicillin, are made from the penicillium mold mycotoxins, which kill bacteria. As a result, the beneficial bacteria of the GI tract can be impacted.

There have been very few human studies related to mold toxicity, so the medical community simply isn't aware of the extent of the issue.

The vast majority of studies about mold and mold toxins are related to animals and animal feed. There has been no real funding or movement towards bringing this work into the human realm: no research, no definitive lab tests, and no human trials for treatments.

What we know from animal testing is that mycotoxins are carcinogenic, hepatotoxic (damaging to the liver), neurotoxic, cardiotoxic, lymphotoxic, and immunosuppressive.[8] They interfere with cellular processes, such as RNA and DNA synthesis, and are therefore cytotoxic (causing cell damage).[9]

Human exposure to mycotoxins occurs primarily through inhalation of air and dust containing mycotoxins, but can also occur through ingestion of contaminated foods, as well as through skin contact with contaminated surfaces.

Food sources of mycotoxins include plant-derived foods that are contaminated with mycotoxins and their metabolites in animal products such as meat and eggs, as well as improperly stored grains. Unfortunately, mycotoxins are resistant to most food-processing methods, including heat.

They are so small (under 0.1 microns) that they bypass mucociliary clearance, the innate defense system in the lungs, and can be absorbed into circulation via the alveoli in the lungs during inhalation, as alveoli are larger, just under 1 micron in size.

Mycotoxins are ionophoric, meaning one end is lipophilic, and the other end is hydrophilic. Because they have the ability to dissolve into fats at one end, and water at the other, they can move through any body tissue, membrane or cell at will.

Health impacts

Mycotoxins' pathogenic effects are multifactorial and can target all organ systems, including the nervous system, urinary system, immune system, endocrine system, reproductive system, and integumentary system, which includes the skin, hair, nails, and glands.

Oxidative stress and inflammation are mechanisms that contribute to mycotoxin-induced toxicity. Mycotoxins have been shown to induce depletion of intracellular glutathione (our master antioxidant in the body), and studies suggest that antioxidants may mitigate the toxic effect of mycotoxins associated with oxidative stress.[10] Mycotoxins activate an inflammatory response in human macrophages (white blood cells that destroy microorganisms), intestinal inflammatory diseases, airway inflammation, and atopic dermatitis. Mycotoxins have been shown to impact micronutrient absorption, distribution, metabolism, and excretion.

Mycotoxins are often neurotoxic, which means they can impact the enteric nervous system in the gut, dysregulating the migrating motor complex.[11] As motility slows, constipation can result. Without regular, daily bowel movements, all toxins are unable to be eliminated effectively and can begin to recirculate, creating greater toxicity.

Very few studies have been conducted looking at the impacts of mold and mycotoxin illness, but those that have been completed show wide-reaching impacts to immune function, neurological concerns, and impaired GI health.

A 2011 study measured IQ scores in 227 children exposed to indoor mold for more than two years. It showed statistically significant IQ deficits of about 10 points in these children. It also showed that longer exposure to indoor mold tripled the risk for IQ scores below the 25th percentile.[12]

Different types of mycotoxins inhibit different detoxification pathways in the liver, which we'll explore in more depth in Chapter 10. When inhaled, mycotoxins are circulated via the bloodstream to the liver where they can cause inflammation and cell damage. Mycotoxins can impair every detoxification pathway in the liver, which then impairs the liver's ability to remove all toxins effectively, contributing to further congestion and recirculation of toxins throughout the body.

One of the few human studies on mold toxicity illness is a 2003 Tufts University study that looked at 100 patients who had been exposed to toxic molds in their homes.

In terms of immune function, they all had immunodeficiencies, which included decreased white blood cell and total lymphocyte counts. Abnormal cell-mediated immunity was identified in 71% of the patients, meaning they had a decreased reaction to infections such as proteus, TB, candida, staph, strep, diptheria, and tetanus.[13] Abnormalities in T and B cells (part of the immune system) were also found in more than 80% of the patients.

Respiratory symptoms were found in 64% of all patients.

Physical signs and symptoms of neurological dysfunction (such as the inability to stand on the toes or walk a straight line with eyes closed) were identified in 70% of patients. Brain CT scans were abnormal in 26 (86%) of 30 patients tested. Objective neuropsychological evaluations of 46 of the patients who exhibited symptoms of neurological impairment showed typical abnormalities in short-term memory, executive function and judgment, concentration, and hand-eye coordination.

GI symptoms that resulted in IBS were found in a quarter of the patients.

Objective abnormal autonomic nervous system tests (heart rate variability) were positive in all 100 patients tested.

It's important to understand that not everyone is equally as susceptible to the impacts of mold. Genetic variations can predispose some of us to mycotoxin illness more than others, and one in four people have the genetic makeup that predisposes them to an increased severity of symptoms when exposed to these mycotoxins. This is why some families can live in the same home together and only one person becomes ill from the impacts of mold.

Women are also more susceptible to mycotoxin illness than men due to a number of factors, including genetic variations and overall toxin burden. Remember the analogy of our toxin "bucket." Every day women come in contact with toxins from makeup, body lotion, shampoo/conditioner, fragrances, and other body care items, in addition to medications such as birth control, additional vaccinations, and even cleaning supplies. While there is a variation for us all – and this by no means indicates that men don't also face a daily toxin burden – women tend to have higher rates of liver dysfunction, which then contributes to the inability to detoxify from mycotoxins when we inevitably come in contact with them. Mycotoxins are also stored in fat cells and women biologically have more fat cells, which means that their burden of stored mycotoxins can climb higher at faster rates.

Symptoms associated with mycotoxin illness:

Eyes, Ears, Nose

- Increased sensitivity to chemicals
- Sneezing and runny noses
- Post-nasal dripping
- Bloody noses
- Nasal polyps
- Swollen lymph nodes
- Sore throat
- Voice changes
- Chronic allergies
- Ear popping
- Ear ringing
- Hearing loss
- Dry or irritated eyes
- Red, itchy, watery eyes
- Sinus inflammation

Respiratory System

- Coughing, wheezing
- Frequent chest colds
- Difficulty breathing
- New asthma diagnosis
- Chronic dry cough
- Burning lungs
- Sensitivity to fragrance
- Chronic respiratory illnesses
- Blood-stained spit or sputum
- Smoke, exhaust or chemical sensitivity

Gut/Digestive System

- Damaged intestinal lining
- Malabsorption of nutrients
- Food sensitivities
- Intestinal inflammation
- Metallic taste in mouth
- Abdominal pain, bloating, cramping
- Diarrhea or constipation
- Nausea and/or vomiting
- Irritable bowels
- Cyclical vomiting syndrome
- Bloating
- Increased gas
- Abdominal cramps or pains
- Ulcers
- Lightning pains
- Food sensitivities or allergies
- Sweet and/or salty cravings
- Food aversions

Brain/Nervous System

- Debilitating brain fog
- Poor focus
- Poor short-term memory
- Headaches
- Confusion
- Sensitivity to light
- Fatigue and lethargy
- Tingling and numbness in hands and feet
- Appetite changes
- Weight changes
- Increased thirst
- Anxiety or depression
- Lightheadedness
- Dizziness
- Slow thinking
- Forgetting words
- Dementia
- Incoordination
- Slow reflexes
- Insomnia
- Neuropathies
- Tremors
- Seizures
- Daytime fatigue
- Poor balance

Urinary System

- Kidney inflammation/bilateral lower back pain
- Overactive or irritable bladder
- Recurrent bladder infections
- Interstitial cystitis
- Incontinence
- Blood in urine
- Kidney disease

Circulatory System

- Spider veins
- Easy bruising and/or bleeding
- Cherry angiomas
- Varicose veins
- Raynaud's syndrome
- Irregular heart beat
- Heart palpitations
- Low or reactive blood pressure
- Low cardio tolerance
- Inability to exercise

Skin/Integumentary System

- Rashes
- Hair loss
- Acne
- Sensitive skin
- Itchy skin
- Burning sensation under skin
- Flushing/redness
- Sensitivity to sunlight
- Peeling or sloughing skin
- Fungal rashes/infections

Immune System

- Increased susceptibility to infections
- Reduced ability to fight acute infections
- Chronic flu-like symptoms
- Intermittent chills and/or fevers
- Long-lasting or recurrent colds
- Chronic or reactivated Epstein-Barr virus (EBV)
- Reactivated previous viral infections
- Frequent herpes outbreaks
- Viral infections becoming bacterial

Musculoskeletal System

- Muscle cramps
- Joint pain
- Bone pain
- Burning muscles
- Arthritis

Reproductive System

- Changes in menstrual cycle
- Estrogen dominance symptoms
- Vaginal yeast or bacterial infections
- Jock itch
- Infertility in both sexes
- Endometriosis
- Dysmenorrhea and amenorrhea
- Premenstrual dysphoric disorder (PMDD)

PART TWO

Restoring Whole Body Health to Support Fertility

Toxicity is one of the driving factors for systemic impacts to our health, both directly and indirectly.

Toxin burden not only disrupts your body's ability to detoxify effectively in key organs such as the liver, but also creates a susceptibility for the overgrowth of pathogens designed to combat these toxins, impairs endocrine function systemically to impair reproductive health, and depletes your body of the minerals and nutrients it needs to function optimally.

Toxicity in the liver creates dysfunction and impairs this vital organ's ability to protect you from toxins long-term, creating a self-fulfilling prophecy where we're unable to remove toxins, and they recirculate and damage tissues slowly over time. Liver dysfunction and heavy metal burden can contribute to hypothyroidism, driving metabolism lower and impairing the ability to replicate embryonic cells effectively.

Many of the toxins we encounter create a terrain in which various pathogenic organisms thrive and overgrow. Glyphosate is metabolized by the Pseudomonas species of bacteria, which can begin to overgrow in the digestive tract, contributing to a wide range of symptoms that burden the immune system, create an upregulated stress response, and impact adrenal, thyroid, and sex hormone function consequently.

We'll discuss these concepts in depth in the coming chapters to help you determine areas that you may need to focus on to rebalance your health to support fertility, but it's important to understand that toxicity is the problem, and it's the most important part of restoring whole body health. If toxicity is not resolved, while any other imbalances can be addressed, it will be impossible to heal fully if exposure to toxins persists.

All of these factors are stress on the body, and when your body is under an immense amount of stress through toxicity, internal demands, nutrient depletions, and poor metabolic function, it will do everything in its power to protect you. Your body makes no mistakes in its infinite wisdom to keep you safe, and unfortunately, reproduction and the associated hormones are the first to be shut off in times of stress for the body.

While overpopulation concerns were rampant for decades, we're now seeing infertility rates expected to grow in a way that may impact the population in a profound way. Population growth from 1950 to 2010 was rapid, with the global population nearly tripling and the U.S. population doubling, but between 2010 and 2050, population growth is estimated to be significantly slower.

To conceive and carry a child means to also birth and raise a child, and with it comes big contributions from the health of the mother, as we pass on everything to our children. If your body is already struggling to support immune function, overloaded with toxins, and running on fumes from deficiencies, it will turn down the dial on conception capacity to protect you in what it perceives to be an unsafe environment for conception.

It can feel overwhelming and impossible to avoid toxins in our modern world. The truth is, it is impossible, and complete avoidance is not the goal. Instead, what you can do is control the controllables, adopt a lifestyle that supports detoxification, and rebalance the impacts on your body to the best of your ability.

While you may currently be thinking about conceiving a child and fulfilling your dreams of being a mother, being aware of these factors and changing the way that you fill your toxin bucket will not only benefit you – it will benefit your future children and protect them from being faced with the chronic diseases that are so common in our society. When we give birth to children who come from mothers who have done their due diligence to detox their bodies, rebalance the resulting health conditions from toxicity, and promote a lifestyle of detoxification by understanding what we are being faced with today, we bring a new generation of health for our children. Current estimates on health indicate that our children are the first generation that will not outlive their parents, but all that can change when we understand what we are up against and take actions in our own homes.

In the coming chapters, we'll explore eight core principles to provide a framework for assessing your toxicity and any impacts to your health that may be negatively impacting fertility. I encourage you to start with supporting drainage and reducing toxicity, as these two core principles are the cornerstone for all subsequent concepts. If this process feels overwhelming, these are the core principles to focus on.

As you explore the impacts of toxicity on mitochondria, gut health, liver function, the thyroid, and nutrient depletions, you'll have symptom assessments to help serve as guidance in determining if these areas of your health may be impacted. In many cases, functional testing is recommended alongside working with a skilled practitioner to interpret your labs. Also included are key strategies for rebalancing these systems on your own when possible.

Because we are consistently exposed to toxicants in our modern world, creating a lifestyle that supports natural detoxification through the concepts in this book will give you the ability to better withstand these exposures while also making critical choices in your home environment.

Chapter 8:

Clearing Your Body of Toxins: The Critical Role of Drainage

> CORE PRINCIPLE ONE: Support drainage pathways as the cornerstone to all detoxification and elimination

Drainage is core to the removal of all toxins and pathogens in the body and essential for wellness. You can think of your drainage pathways as literal drains. When you fill up the sink (or bucket, as in the case of toxins), it must drain out somehow. These drainage pathways are essential for the removal of toxins that our body creates, such as hormones and waste products. When drainage is inhibited, this can result in the recirculation and dominance of hormones such as estrogen and testosterone. The same is true for toxins that we are exposed in our day-to-day lives. What you are not eliminating, you are recirculating.

Figure 8.1

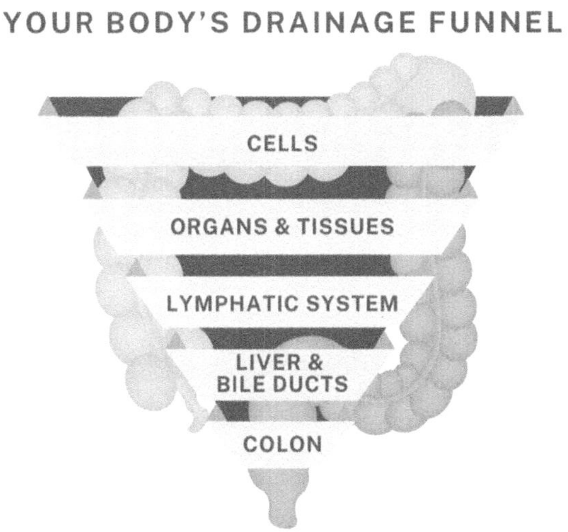

As you'll see in the drainage diagram, the colon is the bottom of the funnel. If this drainage pathway is impaired, in the case of constipation for instance, all other drainage capacity will be impacted. If the colon is working effectively, but the liver and bile ducts are congested, the lymphatic system, organs, tissues, and cells will overflow with toxicity, and so on.

Working from a bottom-up perspective for drainage is crucial for your safety. If the colon is backed up and not eliminating toxins, but you push drainage and detoxification in the liver, toxins will be released with nowhere to go. We'll walk through ways to support each phase of the drainage funnel and additional ways to support drainage systemically, based on where you notice stagnation.

Also of note, when drainage is impaired at the level of the liver and colon, the kidneys, skin, and lungs can be used as a type of "emergency exit" for the removal of toxins. This can result in conditions such as eczema, rashes, psoriasis, acne, urinary tract infections (UTIs), kidney infections, and respiratory issues. If you experience any of these issues, your drainage system is in trouble.

Other symptoms associated with poor drainage:

- Constipation
- Inability to sweat
- Cellulite
- Loss of appetite
- Bloated after meals
- Anxiety & depression
- Mood fluctuations
- Hormonal imbalances
- Weight gain/loss resistance
- Poor memory
- Brain fog
- Chronic fatigue

- Waking up between 1 and 4 a.m.
- Edema & swelling
- Swollen glands
- Yellowish skin
- Acne, rashes, eczema, hives
- UTIs
- Spider veins

The colon

As mentioned, when you take a look at the drainage funnel (Figure 8.1), the large intestine, otherwise known as the colon, is at the bottom. If the colon is backed up, everything upstream from it can become backed up as well. This can happen when you are constipated, which is why daily bowel movements are crucial for the removal of toxins.

If you are not having at least one bowel movement daily, you are constipated. Under ideal conditions, bowel movements are happening between one and three times per day at a normal consistency. I've met women who have experienced constipation for their entire life, typically going 1–2 days without a bowel movement. While this is an incredibly common presentation for women, it is not normal and not something that we would consider healthy.

In more severe cases, I've seen women who are only able to have a bowel movement once every two weeks and are reliant on herbs, coffee, magnesium, and enemas to stimulate a bowel movement. Which brings me to my next point: if you have to use something like coffee every morning to ensure you are having a bowel movement, you are also experiencing constipation.

What should your poop look like to be considered healthy?

Poop and bowel movements are a taboo topic, but the truth is that everyone poops, and as a crucial component in our ability to remove toxins, understanding if we are in an optimal place for colon cleansing is a crucial first step to supporting natural detoxification. Step number one is taking a closer look in the toilet for clues.

Take a look at the Bristol Stool Chart in Figure 8.2. This chart indicates the transit time of stool through the intestinal tract and can help us better understand optimal bowel movement consistency.

Figure 8.2

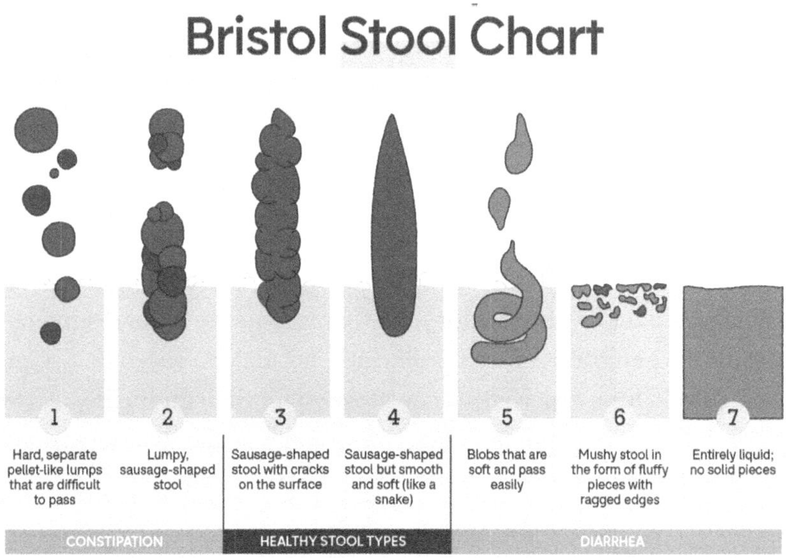

Type 1 and Type 2 indicate constipation and slow transit time, even if that is happening on a daily basis. Constipation can be caused by dehydration, poor diet quality, impaired chemical digestion of food, mineral deficiencies, and pathogenic overgrowths. Gastroparesis, and structural impairments or obstructions, such as the proliferation of endometrial tissues, can also contribute to constipation.

Type 5, Type 6, and Type 7 indicate a faster than optimal transit time, otherwise known as diarrhea or loose stools. This can be caused by food sensitivities, low fiber intake, and pathogenic overgrowths releasing toxins that trigger diarrhea.

Type 3 and Type 4 are considered optimal for intestinal transit time, and while they're not a diagnostic assessment of a healthy gut microbiome, they are a good sign that things are in a good place.

Ways to support colon drainage

It's important to start with dietary and hydration strategies to address constipation. For many, this will be enough to support daily bowel movements, while for others, supplementation may be needed as you continue to address contributing factors for the constipation, such as microbiome imbalances, liver function, and mold.

Assuming that you're consuming adequate water and electrolytes and consuming fiber in your diet, (ideally 2–3 cups of non-starchy vegetables per meal), then you may need to support colon drainage symptomatically. Ensuring regular bowel movement is crucial for healing on every level, and while relying on anything to stimulate a bowel movement is not ideal, it's a crucial step to ensuring you're able to eliminate toxins effectively.

Trace minerals, as well as humic and fulvic acids, can help support not only hydration but also colon drainage, specifically through the electrical charges of electrolytes.

Here are some of the best ways to support colon drainage symptomatically:

Magnesium citrate and magnesium oxide

Both types of magnesium have a laxative effect and stimulate motility to support routine bowel function. Under normal circumstances, one of the key roles of the colon is the reabsorption of water. By using magnesium citrate, the reabsorption of water is inhibited, thus promoting motility at a fast rate and producing a laxative effect. Not everyone tolerates magnesium citrate well, though it is the most bioavailable form of magnesium.

The alternative is magnesium oxide, which stimulates motility without inhibiting the reabsorption of water in the colon. This is best used by anyone who is sensitive to citrate and experiences diarrhea as a result of using it. While magnesium citrate can stimulate a bowel movement in this way, it can also contribute to dehydration, which is not ideal. However, magnesium oxide does not contribute to overall magnesium intake, as this oxygenated form of magnesium serves to stimulate the bowels, but is not absorbed in the same way that other forms of magnesium are.

Ginger

Ginger is a widely used digestive aid, as it is a natural agent that promotes GI motility, preventing food from sitting throughout the digestive tract for long periods of time. Ginger can be added to food, drank as tea, or even utilized in supplement form.

Senna tea

Senna tea contains active ingredients and compounds called anthraquinones, which are sennosides (agents that treat constipation). Most of the research studies on the health benefits of senna focus on its use in the temporary treatment of constipation and other gastrointestinal disorders. Long-term use is not recommended, as it can contribute to dehydration and electrolyte imbalances.

Triphala

Triphala is a polyherbal medicine and has been used in traditional Ayurvedic medicine for centuries. It is a mixture of the dried fruits of three plants native to India: Amala (Emblica officinalis), Bibhitaki (Terminalia bellirica), and Haritaki (Terminalia chebula). Studies show that it is not only effective in the treatment of constipation,[1] but it also reduces gastrointestinal inflammation and repairs intestinal damage.[2]

Water enemas

Enemas are an affordable, at-home version of colon hydrotherapy that can be supportive of relieving stubborn constipation. The most important component of a water enema for ensuring your safety is to use sterilization equipment and distilled water. You can find affordable at-home enema kits in health stores, as well as on mass-market websites like Amazon. You'll find more information and instructions for conducting an enema at home in the following section on the liver.

The liver

The liver and bile ducts are next-highest in the drainage funnel and are one of the biggest sticking points for many women, due to the immense amount of toxins that we ask our liver to filter from our blood on a daily basis. The liver plays a crucial role in converting toxins to water-soluble forms for excretion, and one crucial component of this process is the production and release of bile. This dark-green to yellowish-brown fluid is produced by the liver and aids the digestion of lipids in the small intestine. It is produced continuously by the liver, released into the bile duct, and stored in the gallbladder. After we eat, this stored bile is discharged into the duodenum to assist in the digestion of fats.

Bile is also essential for the conjugation, or binding, of hormones to be removed through the colon via waste (i.e. the stool).

We'll discuss liver toxicity and additional strategies for supporting the liver in Chapter 12, but we want to first discuss how you can support liver drainage and detoxification from a lifestyle perspective, as these will be crucial supports to begin implementing as the foundation for all changes detailed in the coming chapters.

The composition of hepatic bile is 98% water, 0.7% bile salts, 0.2% bilirubin, 0.51% fats (cholesterol, fatty acids, and lecithin), and 200 meq/l inorganic salts.[3] This means that hydration is paramount in the production of bile. If you're dehydrated, especially chronically, bile production will suffer as a result.

Fatty acids are also crucial for the production of bile. Without adequate bioavailable fat in the diet, not only will bile production be inhibited, but the release of bile in the gallbladder will become sporadic, result-

ing in sludgy bile and decreased gallbladder function.
Below, you'll find some of the best ways to support drainage of toxins in the liver:

Castor oil packs
Castor oil packs are an affordable and non-invasive method for supporting liver function and natural detoxification efforts. Castor oil contains a compound called ricinoleic acid, which exhibits anti-inflammatory and analgesic properties.[4] When applied topically, ricinoleic acid penetrates the skin and stimulates lymphatic circulation, aiding in the removal of toxins and waste products from the liver. Ricinoleic acid also reduces inflammation and dysfunction in the liver, thus improving blood flow to the liver to allow it to function optimally.[5]

Castor oil packs are also used to relieve constipation, and this benefit is likely due to the increased production of bile in the liver.[6]

To conduct a castor oil pack at home, follow these steps:

1. Determine what you'd like to use for your "pack." You can use a piece of wool or cotton cloth cut into a rectangular piece around 12 inches by 10 inches, or you can purchase a pack (typically made of organic cotton).
2. Pour approximately 1 tablespoon of organic, cold-pressed castor oil onto your cloth, making sure it is well-saturated.
3. Place the cloth/pack with the castor oil directly on your skin over your liver area, which is located on the right side of your abdomen just under the rib cage.
4. Cover the cloth with plastic wrap or a towel to hold it in place and to prevent oil stains on clothing or bedding. Be sure to wear clothes that you don't mind getting a little oil on.
5. Relax and allow the castor oil pack to remain in place for at least 15 minutes. You can keep the pack placed for up to an hour or even overnight, but start slowly. As you encourage detoxification, it's important to ease into it, especially if you are more sensitive or suspect

you'll be detoxing a lot of toxins. Increase the time duration slowly.

6. Afterward, remove the pack and gently cleanse the skin with warm water and mild soap to remove any residual oil. The pack can be stored in a resealable bag in the refrigerator and reused until it starts to change color. Every couple of days, a small amount of oil should be added to the pack to keep it fully saturated. The castor oil pack should be replaced every two months.

Castor oil packs can be applied daily or at a minimum, three times per week, to support liver detoxification and bile flow.

Coffee enemas

While they may seem fringe even in holistic health, enemas have existed for centuries, with the earliest medical text in existence, the Egyptian Ebers Papyrus (circa 1500 BC), noting the use of enemas to support cleansing.[7] They were mentioned in Shakespeare's work and other worldwide literature, and Native Americans utilized them by using animal products as equipment.[8] John Harvey Kellogg, MD, reported in the Journal of American Medicine in 1917 that in over 40,000 cases of GI disease, only 20 people needed surgery when using enemas routinely.[9] Coffee enemas in particular became more popularized in the 1930s with Max Gerson and the Gerson method of cancer therapy, where he used up to eight enemas per day to help people heal from cancer.[10]

Coffee enemas support the elimination of waste by stimulating the release of bile. The caffeine in therapeutic coffee, also known as green coffee beans, is rich in palmitic acid and theobromine, which are able to open bile ducts to release bile more effectively.

Unfortunately, little research has been done on the mechanisms by which coffee enemas work, but it's believed that the caffeine in the coffee travels through the portal vein in the colon to the liver and gallbladder to release bile. It is also believed the glutathione S-transferase is increased, which aids the body in detoxification.

In the time it takes to hold an enema (roughly 10–15 minutes), the entirety of the body's blood passes through the liver 4–5 times, supporting thorough detoxification of toxins in their journey to exit the body.

To conduct a coffee enema at home, you'll need to collect a few supplies, many of which can be found in health-food stores or in mass markets like Amazon. These options are generally very affordable.

Supplies you will need:

- Enema kit
- A pot with a lid
- Olive or coconut oil for lubrication
- Fine mesh strainer
- Coffee
- Distilled water
- Non-toxic soap
- Glass measuring cup and tablespoon
- Hydrogen peroxide

When choosing an enema kit, you have several options. Glass buckets are non-toxic and will last a lifetime while allowing you to see the liquid emptying, but they are breakable and difficult to travel with. Stainless steel buckets are non-breakable, last a lifetime, and are easy to travel with, but you're unable to see the liquid emptying. Plastic buckets are another option for a non-breakable, travel-friendly enema kit, but they do need to be changed every 3–4 years and can contain toxic plastics. Silicone bags are lightweight and easy to travel with, and you can see the liquid emptying, but they must be changed every 2–4 years, and some people are reactive to silicone. Regardless of the option you choose, be sure to buy a kit with a check valve to prevent backflow into the tubing. This is more hygienic. A clamp for the tubing is also recommended, as it makes controlling the flow of liquid seamless, especially as you learn the process of doing this at home.

To make the coffee for your enema, you'll first want to choose a therapeutic, organic, and mold-free coffee. The cleanest options are those that are air roasted, and the lighter the roast, the more powerful the detox will be. Medium roast is a good starting place for most people. Popular brands include Purelife, Cafe Mam, and Aussie Health. Put 1–2 tablespoons of coffee into 2–4 cups of water in a pot and bring to a boil for 3 minutes, then allow to simmer for 12 minutes. Once done, remove from the burner to avoid water loss. Allow the coffee to cool to a warm temperature (around 99 degrees Fahrenheit), using a thermometer to check the temperature. If you don't have a thermometer, you can put your pinky finger into the solution for at least 10 seconds to determine if it's a comfortable temperature. Then pour the coffee through the strainer into your enema bag or bucket.

To conduct the coffee enema, follow these steps:

1. If possible, have a bowel movement before doing the enema. If you cannot, you might consider doing a water-only enema first, followed by a coffee enema. Prepare your enema coffee solution and pour into your enema bucket or bag. Make sure the tubing is clamped.
2. Open the tubing to allow the coffee to run to the bottom of the tube (and some runs out into the sink or toilet). This releases any air bubbles from the tube. Re-clamp.
3. Find a comfortable place to lie down, such as the floor or bed. Put a towel, plastic sheet, or a "puppy" pee pad (Chux pad) under your hips.
4. Hang the enema bucket 12" to 18" above the surface you will be lying on. The higher the bucket, the faster the flow; however, if it is too low, it won't flow at all.
5. Lubricate the tip well with olive or coconut oil to avoid damaging the tissue, then lie down on your right side with the enema tubing behind you. Insert the lubricated tip three inches into the colon.
6. Open the tubing clamp and allow the coffee solution to flow into the rectum. Be sure to go slowly, as a fast flow can be uncomfortable

and cause cramping. Take your time and let the solution in slowly.

7. When you feel a little full, shut the tubing clamp shut. Withdraw the enema tip or colon tube. Now hold the solution in for 15 minutes, if you can. Try deep breathing if you need to. If you have trouble holding it in, you can keep the enema tip in or you can mix in 1 tbsp organic blackstrap molasses the next time you do an enema to help lengthen the duration. Don't hold longer than about 18 minutes; otherwise, toxins can re-enter circulation and it is counterproductive. You are also more likely to absorb the liquid if you hold too long.
8. Once complete, you may go to the toilet and release the solution.
9. Drink plenty of water afterwards – at least 2–3 liters during the day.

After completing the enema, it's important to clean your equipment each time. Use soap and water in the bucket/bag and run soapy water through the tubes. Rinse the tubes with water afterwards. Then you can pour 1–2 cups of hydrogen peroxide in the bucket and let it run out of the tube to clear any organic matter from the equipment. Once clean, hang the tube and bag/bucket to dry before using it again. Once completely dry, all equipment can be placed in a storage bag.

Coffee enemas can be completed at varying frequencies, but in general, you should consider this 2–3 times per week. Some people find benefits from doing this daily.

The lymphatic system

The lymphatic system is a network of tissues, vessels, and organs that work together to move a colorless, watery fluid called "lymph" back into your bloodstream.

There are four primary functions of the lymphatic system:

- Immune function: The lymphatic drainage system is part of the immune system and allows for rapid identification of pathogens/antigens and the stimulation of an immune response.

- Fluid balance: The lymphatic system helps to maintain extracellular fluid balance, supporting optimal functioning of organ systems. It also absorbs fluid that has leaked outside of the bloodstream, filters it, and then returns it to the bloodstream.
- Detoxification/waste removal: The lymphatic system filters damaged cells and metabolic byproducts via the lymph nodes you may be familiar with. This includes such things as carbon dioxide and the byproducts of cellular oxygen, nutrient, and mineral usage. The lymphatic system then releases these through perspiration, bowel movements, urine, and breathing.
- Nutrient transport: The lymphatic system is also responsible for the transport of lipids (fats) and fat-soluble vitamins absorbed in the digestive tract to other organs/areas of the body.

When the lymph system becomes stagnant, it can impair the ability of any of these key functions to happen seamlessly, but it may also result in swollen lymph nodes, stiffness throughout the body, headache, bloating and digestive issues, fatigue, dry or itchy skin, and swelling (typically in the lower extremities).

How to Support Your Lymphatic System

There are several ways to support healthy lymphatic system function and flow. While some of these approaches are easy to put in place, it can be helpful to choose a few at a time and rotate to see which ones you find most beneficial.

- Hydration and nutrition: Make sure you are drinking high-quality water and eating a diet rich in whole, real foods, ideally organic, and rich in fresh fruits and vegetables. You'll learn more about both of these in Chapter 9. For now, it's important to understand that the lymphatic system is reliant on proper hydration in order to move fluid effectively.
- Limit toxin exposure: Refer to the various sections on reducing toxin exposure in specific areas, including food, water, beauty, home,

air, and clothing to reduce toxin burden on the lymphatic system.
- Movement: Whether you consider your movement "exercise" or are simply able to walk, mechanical movement of fluid supports lymph drainage, as well as overall health and immune function. While stretching, cardiovascular exercise, and strength training all encourage lymph movement, a "rebounder", has been found to be the most effective for lymph drainage. A rebounder resembles a small, single-person trampoline that you can jump on, but the resistance is different compared to a normal trampoline. This bouncing movement and the utilization of gravity have been shown to improve lymph drainage systemically by 15–30 times.[11]
- Lymphatic massage: You might consider seeking out a massage therapist who specializes in lymphatic drainage, or you can consider utilizing some at-home self-massage techniques to support the largest lymph areas throughout the body. Dr. Perry's "Big 6 Lymph Drainage" video is one of the best to help walk you through this process.

You'll note that the top-two layers of the drainage funnel are "cells" and "organs & tissues." While these areas are beyond the scope of this book, it is helpful to address a few other key ways you can support drainage in your daily life.

The kidneys

While water quality is crucial for supporting drainage, ensuring that you are not overhydrating can also be important. In an attempt to support hydration, many women are overhydrating, which is flushing their system without the ability to absorb and utilize the water for hydration.

We want to ensure the right amount of water is being consumed to support kidney function without overburdening the kidneys to detox too quickly, so consuming half of your body weight in ounces is a good starting point, and you can always have more based on thirst levels.

Cherry and cranberry juice are both supportive of kidney function as well, due to the antioxidants and phytonutrients they contain. Consuming 4–8 ounces daily can be beneficial.

The skin

As mentioned, the skin becomes a drainage pathway when the colon and liver are overburdened, but the skin is also the largest organ in the body and has mechanisms by which it maintains health. One of those ways is through sweat.

While sweat might not be something you want to promote, sweating is normal and natural. It's important for the removal of toxins that are being pushed out internally, as well as those that we are exposed to externally.

First, it's important to not utilize any antiperspirants. You won't have to worry about body odor – you can still use a deodorant, but it's important to understand that deodorant and antiperspirants serve two different purposes. We'll discuss more when we dive deeper into personal care products, but you also want to be getting sweaty daily in some capacity. How this is achieved will look different for everyone, such as through daily movement, sitting in the sunshine, or using tools to facilitate sweating. You don't need to be pouring sweat, but perspiration is a great way to ensure open drainage pathways via the skin. Promoting sweat can be a great tool for detoxification.

There's a wealth of research that shows that our skin is able to eliminate toxins, primarily heavy metals like mercury, lead, arsenic, and cadmium, in our sweat.[12][13][14]

Mycotoxins can also be detoxed through the skin, and we're also able to eliminate pesticides from sweat, and interestingly at greater levels than in urine. A 2016 study titled "Human Elimination of Organochlorine Pesticides: Blood, Urine, and Sweat Study,"[15] showed that many pesticides are found in higher quantities in sweat, over serum or urine, indicating that sweating is indeed a significant and important detoxification pathway. The use of a sauna also improves insulin and glucose levels, boosts the NRF2 detoxification pathways, improves mitochondrial function, decreases inflammation, stimulates the production of endorphins, increases oxygen transport, and prevents muscle loss.[16]

Saunas are one of the most effective ways to therapeutically support detoxification through the skin. Infrared saunas are superior to conventional saunas because infrared wavelengths can permeate 2–3 inches into the skin and therefore organs, increasing the circulation of blood vessels and causing the body to release many of the chemicals stored in body fat. However, any form of sauna or sweating is better than nothing at all.

When using a sauna, sessions should fall between 20–30 minutes in length. The benefits triple when going from 2–3 sessions per week to 4–7 sessions per week, so I recommend a minimum of 4 sessions per week, while getting sweaty in other capacities on the other days. For traditional saunas, a temperature range of 176–194 Fahrenheit is ideal, while 110–170 Fahrenheit is ideal for infrared saunas. If you don't have a temperature gauge on your sauna, don't worry about the temperature. Let it heat up, then get in. These sessions can be incredibly relaxing, so they are best done at night but are beneficial at all times of the day.

To be most effective with your sauna sessions, start slowly to ensure you don't experience significant detox reactions. If you feel worse after your sauna session or notice detox reactions (headache, fatigue, digestive upset), you may need to decrease the duration or frequency of use.

Before sauna sessions, ensure that you are properly hydrated with both adequate water intake and electrolytes. Dry brushing your skin before starting your sauna session can also support lymphatic drainage and promote the ease with which you begin sweating.

During your sauna session, use a hand towel to wipe the sweat off as it appears to help prevent any reabsorption of released toxins, and sit on a towel if you're using a public sauna.

After your sauna session, be sure to drink plenty of water to rehydrate, including sodium, which is often lost as a result of sweating. You also need to take a shower immediately to avoid reabsorbing toxins as sweat dries on the skin. A cool or cold shower provides the most benefits and helps to close the pores of the skin following a sauna session, while also supporting the nervous system.

The lungs

Not often thought of as a drainage pathway, the lungs are often a sign of impaired drainage, and supporting the lungs can not only ensure that no pathogenesis exists in these crucial organs, but also supports other systems like the nervous system.

Think about the last time you were sick and had a cough. Often, coughs produce mucous as a way to expel things from the body, such as pathogens that are impacting the respiratory system. This is drainage of the lungs at play.

Most of us are not breathing properly to begin with, and as a result, focusing on breath and proper diaphragm breathing can promote drainage of these organs. Several different styles of breathwork exist, and it's important that you find one that works best for you. No matter what, breathing into the diaphragm, also known as "belly breathing," is crucial for fully expanding the lungs. Most of us are breathing shallowly, only reaching the upper quadrants of the lungs and "chest breathing," which does not stimulate the organs in the abdomen the same way.

Some examples of breathwork methods to consider include box breathing, the 4-7-8 breathing exercises, lion's breath, alternate nostril breathing, and resonant breathing. Exercise can also promote healthy breathwork, especially yoga and exercises that focus on the importance of the breath with movement.

The Role of the Nervous System

When discussing drainage and the ability of our body to naturally regulate toxicant exposure, the nervous system is often one of the most crucial and overlooked components in healing the body as a whole, especially in relation to preconception work. In conventional medicine, there's a significant discontinuity between the head (and mental health) and the rest of the body. While it's becoming more accepted that the gut-brain-axis and proper communication between these two organs are critical in healing gut imbalances, the truth is that nervous system dysregulation is rampant in our society and stands as one of the largest blocking factors for healing every system in the body, with inhibiting factors for conception as well.

It's widely accepted that adverse childhood experiences (ACEs) contribute to negative health outcomes,[17] but those who specialize in nervous system regulation now suspect that big traumas are not the only things impacting our nervous system, mental health, and physical health. To break this down, think about trauma in two main categories: big "T" trauma and little "t" trauma. Big "T" trauma includes those events accounted for in the ACEs research, such as abuse, neglect, and parental divorce. Little "t" trauma, on the other hand, is anything that negatively impacts the way that we perceive the world. Examples can be as simple as someone saying something that hurts our feelings, being picked on at school and it shifting our self-esteem, or not feeling seen or heard. As you can imagine, we all have experienced some type of little "t" trauma.

Any time a person experiences a traumatic event, adrenaline rushes through the body, and the memory is imprinted into the amygdala, which is part of the limbic system. The amygdala holds the emotional significance of the event, including the intensity and impulse or emotion. In his work, The Body Keeps The Score, Bessel Van Der Kolk highlights that traumatic stress is at the root of neuroscience, and that traumatic stress is associated with functional and chemical changes in the emotional part of the brain, the limbic area, and the brain stem.

For example, if you're on a roller coaster, your sensory information is "fear, speed, stress, excitement, not life-threatening." The amygdala can read the emotional significance of the event, as it's a fun ride that you'll be off of in three minutes. The amygdala stores the visual images of trauma as sensory fragments, which means the trauma memory is not stored like a story, but rather by how our five senses were experiencing the trauma at the time it was occurring. The memories are stored through fragments of visual images, smells, sounds, tastes, or touch.

Consequently, after trauma, the brain can easily be triggered by sensory input, reading normal circumstances as dangerous. For example, a red light is no longer a red light; now it's a possible spark. A barbecue had been just a barbecue, but now it sounds like an explosion. The sensory fragments are misinterpreted and the brain loses its ability to discriminate between what is threatening and what is normal.
The front part of our brain, known as the prefrontal cortex, is the rational part where consciousness lives, processing and reasoning occur, and we make meaning of language. When a trauma occurs, people enter into a fight, flight, or freeze state, which can result in the prefrontal cortex shutting down. The brain becomes somewhat disorganized and overwhelmed because of the trauma, while the body goes into survival mode and shuts down the higher reasoning and language structures of the brain. The result of the metabolic shutdown is a profound, imprinted stress response.

The vagus nerve is of utmost importance in nervous system health because it connects the brain to the body, and its primary function is to activate our parasympathetic nervous system, also known as the "rest and digest" state of the central nervous system (CNS). The parasympathetic nervous system facilitates digestion, rest, ease, inner peace, compassion, and connection with others, while the sympathetic nervous system is the "fight or flight" state of the CNS. Unfortunately, most of us are in a constant state of sympathetic dominance due to screen use, a never-ending news feed, long work hours, little play and rest, and not doing things we genuinely enjoy.

Ideally, your nervous system is able to shift between parasympathetic and sympathetic easily, but many of us feel deep discomfort when we begin to shift into parasympathetic mode. For example, when you last had a moment to relax, were you able to enjoy it, or did you feel like you should be doing something productive?

Over time, as you give your body more experiences that stimulate your parasympathetic nervous system, your body learns how to shift with greater ease. A body that is in a sympathetic state consistently comes to perceive this "fight or flight" state as normal, safe, and comfortable. A body that is in a parasympathetic state is able to promote digestion, detoxification, and healthy drainage. When you shift out of patterns that keep you chronically stuck, you will find relief. The more often you find relief, the more your body learns how to go into these patterns and then come out of them. As you practice going in and out of these patterns, you are teaching your nervous system how to be more regulated. Vagus nerve exercises increase your capacity to handle stress and determine how quickly you can bounce back from stressful events.

Here are some of the best ways to support vagal nerve function at home:

- Gargling with water in the morning and evening when you brush your teeth. Aim for 30 seconds to one minute.
- Singing –The louder, the better, as this vibration stimulates the nerve physically and is calming.
- Om-ing – This is the same "om" associated with yoga practice. Sitting in a quiet space, chanting a long "om" provides a vibration around the ears, which will connect to the vagus nerve. A study in the International Journal of Yoga found that chanting "om" was helpful in deactivating certain parts of the limbic system in the brain involved in stress and emotional responses, such as the amygdala.[18]
- Laughing while you watch a funny TV show or movie and actually laughing out loud at the funny parts. Spending time laughing with friends and loved ones has the same effect.

- Eye movement exercises – Lie on your back on the ground, interlace your fingers and bring them behind your head at the base of the skull, keep your head center, and look with your eyes to the right until you sigh, swallow, or yawn, and then repeat on the other side. You may blink during the exercise.
- Cold exposure – You can be brave and do a cold plunge, or you can do short spurts in the shower and alternate from hot to cold, back and forth. The longer you can be in the cold the better, but work your way up in a way that feels right for you.
- Meditating can take many forms and does not have to be long and drawn out, but "contemplative practices," such as meditation and yoga, have been found to bring calm, in part, by activating the vagus nerve. Spend five minutes on an app like Headspace, Calm, or Insight Timer for short guided meditations.
- Emotional Freedom Technique (EFT) is a practice of both verbal affirmation and tapping on certain acupressure points along the meridian system (a traditional Chinese concept). This is a psycho-somatic tool to help us acknowledge our thoughts (which have a chemical impact on our physiology) and to process, both energetically as well as physiologically, the blockages and various chemicals found in the body at any given time. Studies have shown that using EFT or meridian tapping is significantly more effective at reducing cortisol levels in the body than is regular talk therapy.[19]
- Shaking or moving the body, especially in acute moments of stress, helps the body process the stress hormones that are circulating throughout it. All animals, after finding themselves in a stressful situation or in a state of fear, will shake, or certain muscle groups will twitch, as a means of clearing stress hormones from their system. Many of us today tend to "sit and stew" in our stressors, which leads to a chronic exposure to various stress hormones, as we are not actively clearing them from our system. Movement, as we know, is so important for myriad reasons, but can be especially beneficial in times of stress.

We are electric beings and our nervous system is reliant on conductivity to send messages and signals that allow for both voluntary and involuntary actions to occur. Emotions are also "electric" and can become trapped in the body and commonly in specific organs, based on the emotion. Studies show that we consistently feel emotions in certain organs and body parts.[20] For instance, you feel anger in your chest, disgust in your stomach, sadness in your throat and chest, shame in your face, and happiness always feels like a warm hug that encompasses your body. According to Chinese medicine, emotions are narrowed down to five core emotions, with anger being stored in the liver, grief in the lungs, fear in the kidneys, worry in the spleen, and joy in the heart.

Addressing emotions rather than shoving them down inside is the best way to support the movement of these energetic emotions out of our bodies. Methods for addressing emotions include talk therapy, confiding in a friend, having healthy outbursts of emotions when they arise, Mind Body Spirit Release™, or somatic therapy.

Chapter 9
Reducing Exposure Sources

CORE PRINCIPLE TWO: Reduce toxicant exposure to support endocrine function and support your future child's health by reducing toxin burden.

"Let food be your medicine and medicine be your food." – Hippocrates

At the very least, our food should not be a primary source of poison for us. While this might not be possible when eating the standard American diet, there are several choices that are within our control to support reducing potentially harmful exposures to ensure the food we eat is actually nourishing us.

The quality and types of food we consume are fundamental to our health, and yet, in our modern world, protecting our health through food is not as simple as we would like it to be. Nourishment in the United States has turned into a commerce endeavor with few other considerations.

Mass-marketed foods are contaminated with pesticides in an attempt to increase production for farmers and create a better yield, thus producing more money. You've likely found yourself wondering if eating organic produce is really worth the extra cost associated with the label? While the food itself contains the same nutritional value, the real benefit comes from the lack of pesticides and herbicides in organic food, which lowers your total toxin burden.

While we would recommend eating organic produce only, doing so is quite expensive. To reduce your overall toxin exposure, you can focus on eating organic for selected types of produce – those that are recognized for containing high levels of pesticides, also known as the "Dirty Dozen." This list is curated by the Environmental Working Group (EWG) and changes on an annual basis. If you're unable to purchase these produce items in their organic form, you could alternatively choose to avoid consuming them.

In 2023, the Dirty Dozen included:

1. Strawberries
2. Spinach
3. Kale and collard greens
4. Nectarines
5. Apples
6. Grapes
7. Bell peppers
8. Cherries
9. Pears
10. Peaches
11. Celery
12. Tomatoes

Congruently, the EWG releases another list annually known as the Clean Fifteen – a list of the clean produce items that contain very little amounts of pesticides and can be eaten when grown conventionally.

The 2023, the Clean Fifteen list included:

1. Avocado
2. Pineapple
3. Onions
4. Papayas
5. Sweet peas
6. Asparagus
7. Honeydew melon
8. Kiwi

9. Cabbage
10. Mushrooms
11. Cantaloupe
12. Mango
13. Watermelon
14. Potatoes
15. Sweet Corn

Eat quality meat

When it comes to consuming quality animal products, it's not just about the nutritional value of foods and avoiding pesticides. However, you will want to consider the fact that many conventionally raised animals are fed grains that have been sprayed with pesticides that then impact the animal's health and can be transferred to us. Animals also have their own unique toxicant exposures beyond what they eat.

Polychlorinated biphenyls (PCBs) are a family of over 200 industrial chemicals used in things like electrical transformers and capacitors, gas pipelines, and in caulking and other building materials. They have also been used as plasticizers in paints, plastics, and rubber products. Because of mounting evidence showing that PCBs were toxic to humans and wildlife, the EPA banned their manufacture, sale, and use in 1979. However, PCBs tend to accumulate in the sediment found in the silt and mud at the bottom of lakes, rivers, and oceans. As a result, bottom-feeding species of fish and shellfish can often have higher levels when compared to surface-feeding fish.

Consistently, studies are finding PCBs, dioxins, and other persistent organic pollutants (POPs) in both meat and dairy cows. In addition to being persistent, they are also lipophilic, which is why they are found in the fatty tissues of animals. In fact, most exposure of "the average American is due to dietary PBDE intake from meat, then fish and dairy."[1] (PBDE stands for polybrominated diphenyl ethers, which are compounds used as a flame retardant.)

Artificial hormones are rampantly used in the beef and dairy industry, as well as in sheep farming. These hormones are used to promote faster growth and higher milk production in animals and can also lead to an increased risk of cancer in the animals, as well as the humans who eat meat treated in this way. The types of growth hormones used in cattle (most often in the dairy industry) specifically, rBST and rBGH, cause a significant increase in something called insulin-like growth factor 1 (IGF-1). Studies have found an increased risk of breast, prostate, and colorectal cancer associated with higher levels of IGF-1.[2 3 4 5]

Hormones commonly used in beef cattle and sheep include estrogen, progesterone, and testosterone, along with a few synthetics, all of which have the potential to cause endocrine disruption and developmental problems. Animals that are treated with these hormones are prone to higher rates of tissue inflammation and infection, which requires an increase in the use of antibiotics.

Antibiotic use is also rampant in conventional livestock practices, with 80% of all antibiotics sold in 2009 being used for livestock and poultry, according to the Natural Resources Defense Council, and only 20% for human use.

This is where pastured and grass-fed meats really show their worth. Grass-fed beef generally contains less total fat compared to grain-fed beef.[6] Less fat means less space for toxins to accumulate.

Grass-fed beef also has higher levels of omega-3 fatty acids,[7] as well as higher levels of vitamin E, beta-carotene, and conjugated linoleic acid (CLA).[8] Beef is one of the best sources of CLA, a compound that exhibits potent antioxidant activity. Research suggests that CLA is protective against heart disease, diabetes, and cancer, and grass- fed beef contains 2–3 times more of it than grain-fed beef.

When it comes to meat and dairy consumption, the best thing we can do is focus on purchasing organic, grass-fed, pastured animals as much as possible. Organic certification requires that all feed, including the pasture they graze on, be 100% certified organic, meaning the land that organic beef graze on cannot be sprayed with pesticides that are not approved under the USDA organic seal. Additionally, the use of most synthetic medicines and/or hormones is prohibited.[9]

We also need to consider that 100% organic doesn't mean that there are no toxins present. Remember that PCBs and dioxins, for example, are in the environment; they're in the soil and air, so even organically raised animals can have some levels of these in their bodies. But choosing organic will certainly help us to decrease exposures to persistent chemicals, pesticides, hormones, and antibiotics, while increasing the nutrient content food from animals raised this way.

A 2010 article published in the journal Reviews in Obstetrics and Gynecology, stated that "seafood can also contain organic mercury and other harmful toxins (such as PCBs), which could be harmful to the growing fetus. For this reason, the FDA/EPA recommends limiting fish consumption to 2 servings per week. Recent surveys have demonstrated that, despite the FDA/EPA advisory indicating that up to 2 servings of fish are safe in pregnancy, many pregnant women consume little to no fish, thereby potentially depriving the fetus of necessary nutrients."[10] The omega-3 fatty acids found in fish are critical building blocks of the fetal brain and retinas and are required for normal growth and development of numerous organ systems. Numerous studies have shown that low fish consumption during pregnancy can lead to lower IQ and behavioral deficits in children.[11] Not eating any fish out of fear and confusion of what's safe isn't good.

Wait ... don't fish contain high levels of mercury that we want to avoid to reduce overall toxicity? Not all fish contain mercury. In fact, the types of fish highest in omega-3s are the least likely to contain high levels of mercury and other heavy metals. Omega-3s are not only important for conception, but also throughout pregnancy to support neurodevelopment.

Figure 9.1

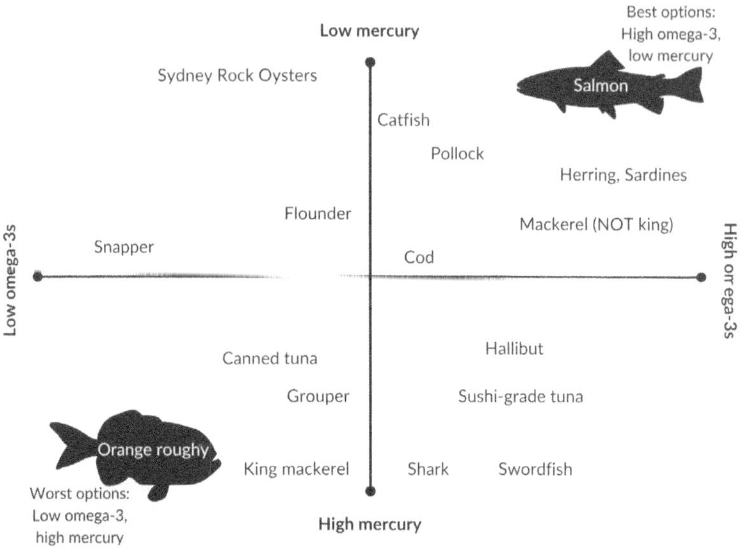

Source: Oyster, E. (2013). *Expecting Better*.

A study published in The Lancet in 2007 looked at prenatal fish consumption and neurodevelopmental outcomes in nearly 12,000 women in the UK. Women who ate less than 12 ounces of seafood a week had a higher risk of having children with suboptimal scores on measures of verbal IQ, prosocial behavior, fine motor skills, and social development.[12] Other studies have explored the link between low omega-3 intake during pregnancy and high levels of depression in the mother.[13]

Water

All life is dependent on water, and as a functional nutritionist, I know that most of us are chronically dehydrated. While increasing water intake is a crucial component of promoting health in every cell in the body – as many systems are reliant on adequate hydration to function properly – most of us aren't thinking about the quality of our water as a key component of our foundational health.

In the United States especially, most of us feel that we are being supplied clean water that is tightly regulated by government agencies to keep us safe, but that belief couldn't be farther from the truth.

As we've discussed the various toxicants that can be driving fertility concerns, you may have noticed that you're exposed to many toxins, such as metals, chemicals, and radioactive substances through drinking water.

But tap water is purified for our consumption, right? To answer this, let's briefly discuss how the tap water that comes out of your sink comes to be.

There are four primary phases of water treatment, beginning with coagulation and flocculation, which are terms used to describe the chemical treatment of sewage water and other water sources that serve to clump particles together for removal. Think of this as the "large particle" screening from water.

Next in the process is sedimentation, which is where the particles are allowed to settle to the bottom of the water in a holding tank. This is followed by filtration, where dust and particles are filtered out of the water down to 1 micron in size. For reference, an atom of lead is 154 picometers in size, which is the equivalent of 0.000154 microns.

The last step in the process is disinfection, where chlorine, fluoride, chlorinates, and chlorine dioxides are added to remove any microbes from the water. These disinfectants are never removed from the water before it reaches your tap, and as we've discussed, these chemical reagents have health impacts of their own.

But tap water purification takes care of everything else, right?

According to the U.S. Geological Survey (USGS), pharmaceuticals are frequently found in tap water due to human excretion, as well as by being flushed down the toilet. In a study conducted by the USGS in 1999 and 2000, measurable amounts of one or more medications were found in 80% of the water samples drawn from a network of 139 streams in 30 states.[14] The pharmaceuticals identified included antibiotics, antidepressants, blood thinners, heart medications (ACE inhibitors, calcium-channel blockers, digoxin), hormones (estrogen, progesterone, testosterone), and painkillers.

One study found that of 159 samples analyzed, 83% were found to contain plastic particles, with the largest density of plastics being found in samples collected in North America.[15] Another study showed that an average of 325 plastic particles were found in a liter of bottled water, as compared to 5.5 plastic particles per liter of tap water.[16] While the tap water levels are less than we would be exposed to from bottled water (naturally, since we know that plastic containers readily leach into the water they contain, at increased temperatures), it's still not zero plastic exposure via tap water.

A study conducted by Consumer Reports in 2011 showed that 35% of tap water samples contained per- and polyfluoroalkyl substances (PFAS), while 8% contained arsenic, and a whopping 98% of samples contained measurable amounts of lead.[17] As we discussed earlier, radioactive substances that include radium and uranium are also found in the tap water in nearly every state in the United States.

Pathogens are an ongoing problem with tap water consumption, as well. The CDC warns of a number of different bacterial, viral, and parasitic pathogens that are known to be present in tap water and provides suggestions such as boiling your tap water before use.[18] They cite sewage overflows, sewage systems that are not working properly, polluted stormwater runoff, or agricultural runoff as possible contributing sources for the contamination of the tap water supply. In the last 30 years, multiple researchers have found parasitic eggs in tap water[19] that have not been removed by typical disinfection methods.

Tap water is often contaminated by agricultural runoff, and the primary concern here is the contamination of pesticides, fertilizers, and other industrial chemicals used in conventional farming. According to the EWG, America's farmlands and rural regions bear the brunt of the harm in terms of consuming runoff from these agricultural chemicals.[20] An 85-mile stretch of land along the Mississippi River is referred to as "Cancer Alley" due to the high levels of cancer and other health conditions in these areas, stemming from the presence of petrochemical plants and the influx of contamination to tap water from the agricultural runoff that is predominant in this area.[21]

It's for these reasons that I'll sternly refer to tap water as "infertility water." If there is one thing you change about your exposure to toxins as a whole to make the greatest impact, let it be to choose a better quality water source.

If you're interested in learning more about what's in the water in your area, you can search your zip code in the Environmental Working Group's water database, which allows you to conduct searches for contaminants that include heavy metals, industrial chemicals, and other water-soluble toxicants. Here you'll find not only the legal limit of each contaminant, but you'll also see the EWG's health limit, as well as the amount found in your own drinking water.

As recently as 2023, the EPA proposed new guidelines to limit drinking water from toxic "forever chemicals" known as PFAS, targeting six well-known variations of PFAS, including PFOA, PFOS, PFNA, PFHxS, PFBS, and GenX.[22] However, we know that it takes, on average, 17 years to implement new health and medical research.[23]

Before you run to the supermarket to buy bottled water, you'll want to know that most bottled water is just tap water – in fact, 64% by most estimates.[24] This means you'll pay a premium to drink the same water you're getting out of the kitchen tap, in most cases.

In addition to the quality of the water you're getting in bottled water, these bottles are often transported and stored in high-temperature facilities that increase the temperature of the plastic the water is contained within, increasing the likelihood of plastics leaching into the water itself. A study that analyzed samples taken from 259 bottled waters sold in several countries found that 93% of them contained "microplastic" synthetic polymer particles.[25]

Fortunately, dirty and plastic-contaminated water aren't your only options for your daily, routine water source. While there's a time and place to have bottled water, such as while traveling, investing in cleaning your water may be one of the best things you can do to lower your total toxin exposure.

Bad, Better, Best

Bad	Unfiltered tap water
Okay	Carbon filtration
Better	Reverse Osmosis
Best	Distillation

Think of water quality on a sliding scale. Improving the quality of the water you drink should be a foundational priority, but know that it also comes with a significant investment. To help you move in the right direction, you can choose an option that is better than what you're currently drinking.

Carbon filtration

Most common water filtration systems utilize carbon filters, including your refrigerator and many pitchers. They utilize carbon filters usually derived from coconut shells or coal and utilize pores in the carbon. These porous chunks of carbon are activated through heat or chemicals to absorb contaminants and make water "purified" or "filtered" for consumption.

Carbon filters are a significant improvement from unfiltered tap water and can remove numerous contaminants, including phosphates, chlorine, pharmaceuticals, pesticides, and lithium, to name a few, but carbon filters are only effective to a certain extent. They're unable to remove many harmful compounds such as nitrates and arsenic, of which carbon filters can only reduce up to 70%.

Reverse osmosis

Reverse osmosis (RO) is a process by which a solvent passes through a porous membrane in the direction opposite to that for natural osmosis, when subjected to a hydrostatic pressure greater than the osmotic pressure.

Reverse osmosis is capable of removing up to 99% of the dissolved salts, particles, colloids, organics, bacteria, and pyrogens from the feed water. This being said, an RO system should not be relied upon to remove 100% of bacteria and viruses. Reverse osmosis filters excel at removing heavy metals due to their efficient filtration mechanism. The microscopic pores of the membrane effectively capture much smaller particles, ensuring that heavy metals are effectively removed from the water supply.

However, it's important to understand that the efficiency of reverse osmosis filters is largely dependent on the amount of contaminant contained in the water you are trying to filter. For example, if your water has 30 mg/L of nitrate, reverse osmosis would be able to reduce that to 3.5–2.5 mg/L. However, if your water contains 100 mg/L of nitrates, reverse osmosis would only be able to reduce the amount of nitrates to 15–10 mg/L. This means that while reverse osmosis is more effective than carbon filters at removing certain, more dangerous contaminants, it is only effective on some amounts of these contaminants.

Distillation

A water distiller works by mirroring the Earth's natural hydrologic cycle, the process by which rain is created through evaporation. First, heat from the sun evaporates water from the surface, bringing it into the atmosphere. Under colder temperatures, the water is condensed and eventually falls to the ground. A water distiller works the same way, where heat is applied to the boiling tank's source water (which can be your tap water), until it becomes steam. This steam is then condensed and the condensation is collected for consumption. In essence, the water is removed from the contaminants rather than the contaminants being removed from the water.

A water distiller can remove arsenic, nitrates, lithium, pesticides, fertilizer, and pharmaceuticals, as well as radioactive chemicals like uranium. The boiling process kills microorganisms such as bacteria and viruses.[26]

Figure 9.2

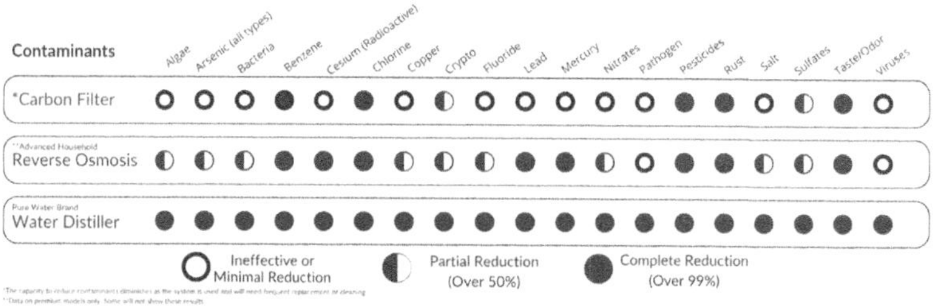

I recommend choosing a distillation option as the best of the best for the removal of all toxins from your water supply. However, purchasing water stored in plastic jugs might not be optimal.

Instead, you can find a local water delivery service for distillation or reverse osmosis water, and it will often come in a hard plastic jug. You can inquire further about the type of plastic used, how jugs are stored, how long they contain water before delivery, and ask other questions to determine possible exposure to see if it's a good fit for you. This tends to be more affordable than the alternative, which is installing your own system in your home. There are several reverse osmosis and distillation systems available on the market at a variety of different price points and with varying space considerations. For instance, you can often find a water pitcher that does either reverse osmosis or distillation (alongside the components to complete these processes), or you can find a whole house system for either option. This allows you to find the best option for your family.

With both reverse osmosis and distilled water, it's essential to replenish the water with minerals. As we'll discuss in more depth in our dietary recommendations, electrolytes are a crucial component of hydration to ensure cellular hydration rather than simply flushing the system of water it is unable to utilize. Consuming distilled water in particular long-term, without adding minerals back into the water, can be detrimental to the mineral status in your body.

Air

According to the National Human Activity Pattern Survey, conducted by the EPA, in the U.S., we spend approximately 87% of our time indoors, and as you can see, almost 69% of our lives in our own homes.[27] As such, the majority of our exposure to environmental toxins is occurring while we are safely within our own homes.

Much of this is due to the recirculation of air in homes that are designed to be airtight and a society that does not properly respect the need for fresh air and air flow. In your home, you're likely coming into contact with PFAS, parabens, VOCs, and flame retardants, at a minimum.

In an analysis of the contaminants in home dust, flame retardants are commonly found in 95–100% of homes due to being sprayed on a number of different surfaces like rugs, furniture, and mattresses to prevent the risk of home fires.[28] A study by the Silent Spring Institute found that of the 16 California homes they tested, 100% had measurable levels of multiple flame retardants in them – 62 different compounds in total.[29] Fifty percent of the samples from that study had over 41 different chemical flame-retardant compounds, including a chemical called brominated tris, which was banned from children's pajamas in 1977 due to its carcinogenicity.[30]

Multiple studies have found that due to commonly playing on the floor, children have higher levels of flame retardants in their bodies when compared to adults.[31] Additionally, another study produced by the EWG in August of 2014 found that in some cases, children had five times the blood levels of flame retardants as their mothers.[32]

Many flame retardants activate what is called the PPAR-y receptor gamma, the primary regulator of fat cell development, which can result in more fat creation as well as a decrease in bone formation. Activation of this receptor drops it into the category of an obesogen, defined as a chemical that can trigger metabolic disruption leading to weight gain or other metabolic conditions.[33]

These flame retardants are also endocrine disruptors and can mimic estrogen[34] in addition to affecting the thyroid.[35] [36] They're also reproductive toxins,[37] with exposure leading to ovarian changes[38] and decreased sperm counts.[39] [40] It's for this reason that air quality is incredibly important, in addition to considering the materials that we bring into our home environment.

When dusting, it's important to not use feather dusters, which simply push and blow dust around, but to "wet dust" and/or use cotton or microfiber cloths that can then be laundered. Implementing a quality air filter that goes beyond the large particle collection of your HVAC system is another way to significantly reduce exposure and recirculation of various toxins in your home. Ideally, you also have a filtration system that accounts for mold and mycotoxins. Mold spores can be released into the air, and when air is stagnant (no open windows), we are more exposed to high levels of mycotoxins in all environments. Considering that most of us spend most of our day at home, filtering the air in our homes can be one of the best steps toward ensuring the mitigation of mycotoxin exposure. When looking for an air filter, look for HyperHEPA, ionizing, or incinerating filters.

In the kitchen

It's time to take a look in your kitchen and decide which items you need to ditch to support your fertility.

Focusing on plastics is a good place to start. The goal is to drastically reduce the negative effects of plastics like BPA and PVC in your home. First, let's review how plastics can migrate easily in a number of environments, even if you may have not realized this before now.

Think about a tupperware container that was crystal clear when you bought it, but is now dull, foggy, and scratched. The surface has become scratched and worn down, whether from scrubbing, going through the dishwasher, or from grinding hard objects against it (like a fork). As this happens, small pieces of the plastic have been lost.

Acidic foods like citrus, tomatoes, or vinegar can increase the rate at which those plastic molecules shed. This occurs so consistently that studies looking at chemical migration from materials often use acetic acid in the lab to provoke leaching. At some point, you've probably had a tupperware container that you were unable to get clean after tomato sauce was stored in it, tinting the plastic orange. No matter how much you wash it, soak it, or scrub it, the orange tint won't come out.

Tomato sauce is the perfect storm of factors in relation to plastic migration: heat, oil, and acidity. When the hot, oily, acidic sauce comes in contact with the plastic food-storage container, the physical lines between the plastic and the food become blurred, and the result is that some of the orange pasta sauce migrates into the physical structure of the plastic. What you're seeing is pasta sauce inside the plastic. It's not on the plastic; it's in the plastic.

The inverse of this is that you're also going to end up with plastic molecules in your sauce.

Never cook food in plastic containers in the microwave. You might even go as far as skipping the use of the microwave altogether, as it's been shown to degrade the nutritional value of food.[41] In addition to keeping plastics out of the microwave, you shouldn't store hot, acidic, and fatty foods in plastic containers for any reason, as there is an increase in migration of plasticizers into these types of foods.[42]

Since plastics are chemically attracted to fatty substances, and therefore accumulate in higher amounts in high-fat content foods stored in plastics, you'll also want to be mindful of the container that holds the following types of products: Oils, salad dressings, mayonnaise, or any other high fat food should ideally never be purchased in plastic bottles. Instead, glass jars are best for these types of fatty foods.

If you have plastic containers in your home, I'd encourage you to at a minimum check for the resin indication code on the bottom of the container. You can do this for all plastic containers including tupperware, condiment bottles, etc. Don't buy anything that comes in a #3 plastic container and ditch anything in your kitchen that already contains this plastic.

In the kitchen, we encounter Styrofoam mainly in the form of Styrofoam food packaging, including egg cartons, takeout containers, and trays for meat and cheese, which are then wrapped in phthalate-containing cling film. Styrofoam is also found in to-go coffee and tea cups. While we're unlikely to experience any meaningful exposure to styrene from an egg carton, we are far more likely to be exposed to styrene that has migrated into foods, especially when they are high in fat and hot when put into the container.[43] This is very common among food for takeout. Styrene migration from Styrofoam is dependent on the fat content and the temperature of the food, so putting hot food into a takeout container or hot beverages into foam cups is going to increase leaching of styrene.[44] When possible, avoid purchasing foods that come in Styrofoam containers and limit takeout that comes in these types of containers.

Styrofoam cups and food packaging are the largest sources of ingested styrene.[45] Despite that, nearly all the data on exposure to styrene has been done on those impacted through smoke inhalation. Exposure to styrene causes oxidative damage and depletes glutathione levels.[46]

Why BPA-free doesn't mean safe

In light of the negative health outcomes associated with bisphenol A (BPA), many companies have shifted towards using "BPA-free" as a label to indicate the safety of their plastic products. Technically, yes, these BPA-free products may not use BPA, but most of the time they do use the chemically similar compounds, BPS or BPF. A 2015 study on BPA and BPS in the journal Endocrinology stated that "BPA-free plastic products are not necessarily safer than products containing BPA."[47]

To be completely safe, skip the use of plastics and plastic containers, when you can. Glass containers are far cleaner and completely safe for the storage of all types of foods, regardless of their temperature, and are even safe for reheating foods. The biggest downside to these types of containers is that they are susceptible to breaking more easily. Consider swapping your tupperware for glass containers, (a plastic or silicone lid is okay as long as it's not touching the fatty or warm food content), and switch to glass or ceramic cups and drinking containers (such as water bottles).

To reduce the health risk of Teflon and other PFAS, it might be time to update your kitchen cookware to include healthier, non-toxic options. This will include all pans, pots, and cooking sheets that have non-stick properties.

Enameled cookware, sometimes called porcelain enamel, is made by fusing powdered glass to a substrate like cast iron. These types of cookware do not leach unless the enamel has been chipped off, exposing the pan underneath. However, if the pan itself is cast iron or stainless steel, there isn't a toxicity issue. While enamel isn't a non-stick surface, it's a "less stick" surface when used correctly.

Enameled cast-iron cookware, like those from Le Creuset and Lodge, are the most popular, but large retailers often sell other brands.

Cast iron has been used to cook foods for centuries, and if cared for, will last multiple generations, if not forever. A well-seasoned pan is essentially non-stick. The seasoning on cast iron is formed by fat polymerization, which in essence creates a strong but thin inert layer. This layer can be destroyed by the cooking of acidic foods, like tomato sauce. For this reason, you'll want to cook acidic foods in enameled or stainless steel cookware.

Cast iron cookware has excellent heat retention qualities and can easily go from stovetop to oven. The two biggest downsides to cast iron are that it can be heavy and difficult to work with, and more importantly, the iron can actually leach from the cookware into your food. For most people, the small amount of iron that can leach into foods isn't a problem, and if someone has low iron, it can actually be a great way to easily add iron to the diet. However, people with known heavy metal issues, hemochromatosis, or excess iron will want to be mindful of cast iron use. Proper seasoning of cast iron can also reduce the amount of iron that leaches into food.

Similar to cast iron, carbon steel is another non-toxic, lightweight option for cookware. Carbon steel still needs to be seasoned and cared for properly. Carbon steel is primarily used to make frying pans and woks, but not pots. Similar to cast iron, carbon steel is not recommended for cooking acidic foods.

Stainless steel is one of the most durable cookware options that is readily accessible and can last a lifetime. It's one of the more costly cookware options, but it's suitable for any kind of cooking. Stainless steel is an alloy, a mixture of metals, and the cookware often contains a small percentage of both nickel and chromium, both of which have the potential to leach in very small amounts. For most people, this is not a concern. Those with heavy metal issues may not want to use stainless steel, due to the minor amount of leaching, but for the average person, stainless steel is an extremely safe surface to cook with.

Roasting pans and baking sheets can also be made out of stainless steel, while traditional options for these are typically aluminum or non-stick coated. Throw out the old ones and invest in quality products to reduce toxicity in your food.

Tempered glass is one of the most inert and safe cookware materials. Tempered glass will not crack as long as you're not cooking at extraordinarily high temperatures. Glass bakeware like brownie pans, loaf pans, casserole dishes, and pie pans are easy to find and are fully non-toxic. The downside to glass, of course, is that it can break, but it's generally not very expensive to replace.

Personal care items

A study conducted by the EWG found that women use an average of 12 personal care products containing 168 unique chemical ingredients, every single day. Men use about 6, which contain about 85 chemicals, each day. Screening the products that you use for personal care can make a huge difference in reducing toxin burden. This includes anything that you put on your body, which can be quite the monumental task to undertake.

Rather than feeling like you need to throw out everything you own and replace them today, you might instead take a gradual approach and slowly make changes to products as you run out of them. However, if you want to do a complete purge, I support your efforts and enthusiasm. A gradual approach tends to be less overwhelming, as well as more cost-effective, since you don't have to purchase everything all at once. I recommend the gradual method for making all changes in toxic products (personal products, household cleaners, and cookware). Another approach to consider is first removing products that go directly in or on your body first (as outlined in the list below), then consider removing products that are absorbed into your body but not intended for use on the body.

When thinking about personal care products, you'll want to consider all of the following:

- Shampoo and conditioner
- Body soap
- Shaving cream or gel
- Lotions and moisturizer
- Facial cleansers
- Dry shampoo and all other hair products
- Makeup (mascara, eyeshadow, lipstick, concealer, foundation, eyeliner)
- Deodorant
- Perfumes
- Sunscreen
- Nail polish and polish remover
- Hair dyes
- Menstrual products (tampons, pads, liners, period underwear)
- Hand soap
- Waxing products

Keep in mind that this is certainly not an exhaustive list, as personal care varies from person to person, but it should provide a good starting point to get you thinking about the products that may secretly contain toxins that are detrimental to your fertility.

There are a number of free tools available to help you navigate which of your products are safe to keep and which you should swap for cleaner options. For instance, the EWG Healthy Living app is free to download and provides a database of products that rates their ingredients; however, it may have data gaps due to the lack of research on some ingredients. Another database is Made Safe, which screens for thousands of ingredients from authoritative "red lists" from around the world, to ensure that no ingredient is a known behavioral toxin, carcinogen, developmental toxin, endocrine disruptor, flame retardant, GMO, heavy metal, neurotoxin, high risk pesticide, reproductive toxin, toxic solvent, or harmful VOC. The Think Dirty app is another free app that rates products and allows you to scan the barcode of products to look up information about the product and any known harmful ingredients.

These apps and databases are not without errors and discrepancies at times, but they can certainly be useful for screening a wide number of products in your home to determine their safety and help you look for better options. You can even use these resources while looking for new products in the store to get an instant idea about their safety.

Before we dive into what to look for in personal care products, it's important to make an important distinction between "penetration" and "absorption." Although these two terms are often used interchangeably, they don't actually mean the same thing.

Penetration happens when a chemical makes it all the way down to the bottom layer of the skin. There is no vascular system within the epidermis, so things that penetrate the skin don't ever reach the bloodstream. On the other hand, absorption happens when a chemical makes its way through all the layers of the skin, into the dermis, which does have a vascular system, and therefore makes its way into circulation in the body.

Many personal care products contain ingredients, referred to as penetration enhancers, that can alter the absorption rate of other chemicals present. Occlusives like silicones create a seal over the skin, which can increase penetration of ingredients that may lead to absorption. Surfactants and solvents can similarly disturb the oil balance of your skin in a way that can increase penetration and/or absorption.

To avoid phthalates most commonly used as fragrance, always avoid anything containing fragrance or perfume. Parabens will be listed on ingredient labels. You'll want to look for any word ending in "paraben."

The key ingredients of concern, outside the fragrances and parabens, are aluminum-based compounds that are primarily found in antiperspirants. Deodorants are intended to simply mask odor and are therefore classified as a cosmetic by the FDA – this is where you'll find heavy use of those fragrances (phthalates).

Antiperspirants on the other hand are classified as a drug by the FDA because they perform a biological function to prevent sweating, and it's the aluminum in these products that are responsible for that process. Aluminum salts are able to stop or significantly reduce the amount of perspiration that's produced under the arms by reacting with your sweat to form a gel plug within the sweat gland itself, essentially blocking any sweat from coming out. These gel plugs also contribute to impaired lymphatic drainage in the underarms where major lymph nodes are located and can contribute to clogged pores in the underarm.

Those yellow stains on white shirts? We can thank the aluminum ingredients in antiperspirant for those. Aluminum reacts with sweat and stains clothing, so it's not the product itself that's ruining the clothes, but the way that the product is interacting with our body chemistry.

Remember that aluminum is recognized as a neurotoxin[48] and is linked to oxidative stress and mitochondrial dysfunction.[49]

A 2001 study found that only a small amount of aluminum was absorbed after a single application of antiperspirant – about 2.5% of the amount that's typically absorbed by the gut.[50] However, this study looked at only a single application without taking into consideration that these products are used daily, sometimes multiple times per day. Another study, this one from 2012, found that significantly more aluminum is absorbed from "stripped skin," i.e., freshly shaved skin.[51] It's been well-established that estrogen can play a significant role in the development and progression of breast cancer, so the ability for the cocktail of estrogen-mimicking compounds in antiperspirants being applied to the skin to migrate into breast tissue is definitely concerning. Aluminum has been measured in breast tissue at higher levels in the outer upper quadrant than in the inner ones, and of course, the outer quadrant of the breast is closest to our underarms, where we are applying antiperspirant. Based purely on the presence of aluminum in antiperspirants, these are products that we should not be using, and switching to a product that does not contain aluminum or fragrance can help reduce the absorption of these toxicants.

Many natural deodorants are now available and include different essential oils in place of fragrance, different absorbent ingredients, and oil or fat to hold it all together. Common ingredients include tea tree and lavender essential oils, baking soda, arrowroot, or corn starches, along with bentonite or zeolite clays, and oils like coconut, shea, cacao butter, or a combination of those.

Transitioning from a traditional antiperspirant can be challenging if you're used to having dry armpits, you have strong body odor, or you're self-conscious about sweating. Your body odor is often a reflection of your diet, with a 2006 study finding that eating red meat made body odor smell less attractive.[52] This doesn't mean that you should avoid red meat consumption, but diet can certainly play a role in body odor, and the effect is often worse before it gets better when detoxing from traditional antiperspirants. As we discussed earlier, sweating is incredibly normal and healthy for detoxification efforts in the body. While it's not socially accepted, sweating is something that you don't want to prevent. Of note, molybdenum deficiency plays a role in the presentation of strong body odor, and heavy metals such as aluminum displace minerals in the body, including molybdenum.

Nail polish is another personal care item to consider swapping out to promote fertility, as many traditional nail polishes contain solvents like benzene, ethylbenzene, and xylenes (collectively called BTEXs), which are associated with greater risk for reproductive problems. Authors of a 2017 study on BTEX chemicals found that they can "target ovarian follicles, corpus luteum, oocytes, embryos, oviducts, ovarian cycles, fertility, and the viability of offspring."[53]

These BTEX chemicals are referred to as "the toxic trio," and starting in 2006, a shift began to occur where top brands of nail polish began marketing themselves as free of these toxins. They are unfortunately not the only toxic chemicals that are relevant here. While the toxic trio are the chemicals in nail polish that have received the most attention, they are by far not the only ones.

Water-based and solvent-based nail polish are fundamentally different from one another at a chemical level. Regular solvent-based nail polish is made from nitrocellulose dissolved in volatile solvents such as butyl acetate, ethyl acetate, or even toxic toluene. Regular nail polish is in the form of a solution, meaning that the nitrocellulose is evenly distributed throughout the liquid solvents. When regular nail polish is painted onto nails, the solvents quickly evaporate and leave behind a hard film of nitrocellulose. Regular nail polish can later be removed by reversing this process. Nail polish removers containing the same or similar solvents as regular nail polish once again dissolve the nitrocellulose and lift it off of your nails.

In contrast, water-based nail polish is made out of an acrylic polymer emulsion. A polymer is simply a substance that has a molecular structure consisting of repeating units. The fact that it is an emulsion means that the tiny particles of acrylic are suspended in water. However, the acrylic polymers are not actually dissolved in the water. After the water-based nail polish is painted onto nails, it slowly dries. The water gradually evaporates into the air or soaks into the nails. The tiny acrylic polymer molecules touch each other and join into longer polymer chains. These bonds hold the acrylic polymers together much more tightly than the nitrocellulose in regular nail polish is held together. Water-based nail polish that has fully cured cannot simply be dissolved with mild solvents the way that regular nail polish can. Instead, the bonds of the polymer chains must be broken. This is why water-based nail polish that has been worn for a long time can be difficult to remove."[54]

Water-based polishes are recommended because they don't have any of the toxic solvents that are used in traditional nail polish, and performance-wise, they come pretty close to what we've become accustomed to. They do take much longer to dry and need to be changed more often so they don't become really difficult to remove.

In addition, water-based polishes can actually be better for your nails because they don't strip the natural oils, like solvent-based polishes do. Some water-based polish brands that are out there are Scotch Naturals, Acquarella, Honeybee Gardens, and Piggy Paint.

Household products

As we've discussed, there are many household products that are traditionally made with harmful, toxic, and downright dangerous chemicals to support cleaning and sanitation efforts in your home. But products don't need to be toxic to be sanitary, and there are many easy things you can implement to allow easy cleaning, without buying into the marketing that tells you that stronger is always better.

What you may not realize is that most cleaning products in our home contain mostly water and similar chemical formulations. We certainly don't need a different spray for every room of the home, but with marketing messages highlighting that a product "kills 99.99% of germs, disinfects, and deodorizes," it's easy to buy into the notion that more is better for us.

While most people understand that looking at ingredient labels for food is important, many of these same people are not checking the ingredients of their cleaning products. To be fair, not all cleaning product manufacturers are being exactly forthcoming with their ingredient lists. For example, according to the website for the abrasive cleanser Comet, 7 ingredients are used in their formulation, but according to a study done in 2009 by the EWG, this product released 146 different air contaminants, including chloroform, benzene, and formaldehyde.[55]

What follows is an overview of some of the top things to avoid using in your household cleaners.

Bleach, also known as sodium hypochlorite, is a chlorine-based chemical that is a broad-spectrum antimicrobial and oxidizer. A 2008 article in Environmental Science & Technology found that the use of chlorine bleach-containing household products can react with soaps and surfactants to produce halogenated VOCs like carbon tetrachloride, a probable human carcinogen and a powerful greenhouse gas that was banned for household use by the FDA.[56] Carbon tetrachloride is used in animal studies to induce toxicity and is known to be toxic to the liver and kidney. This chemical also depletes glutathione, which is essential for proper detoxification.[57] Household bleach is often used in places where it will do more damage than good, for example, when trying to whiten mold or mildew on bathroom grout. It's used in the mistaken belief that it will kill the mold and remove the discoloration at the same time.

Unfortunately, bleach is unable to kill the roots of the mold on a porous material, which means that while you may see the mold removed on the surface, it can cause mold to grow deeper into the porous material. Furthermore, bleach is 90% water, which provides moisture for mold to continue to grow. From a more immediate perspective, disturbing and killing mold on the surface results in the release of spores and mycotoxins into the air, which can make those who are already ill as a result of mycotoxins even worse.

Glycol ethers are solvents that are used in degreasing products, including a wide range of cleaning products. The most common type of glycol ether used in household cleaners is 2-butoxyenthanol. The types of products that often contain 2-butoxyethanol are glass cleaners, all-purpose cleaning sprays, and any cleaner intended for degreasing.

According to the EPA, short-term exposure to 2-butoxyethanol at high levels can cause pulmonary edema and severe liver and kidney damage.[58] The Agency for Toxic Substances and Disease Registry indicates that this chemical is linked to reduced fertility and low birth weight and can cause birth defects in animals.[59]

Methylisothiasolinone (MIT) and methylchloroisothiazolinone (CMIT) are commonly found in liquid detergents, including laundry products, as well as a number of personal care products. MIT and CMIT are widely used preservatives. Laundry detergents also often contain nonylphenol ethoxylate (NPE), which is a surfactant and wetting agent that helps water penetrate into the fibers of clothing. NPEs are endocrine-disrupting chemicals.[60]

On the topic of laundry, not only are detergents often toxin-containing, but so are fabric softeners and dryer sheets. According to the EWG, fabric softeners and dryer sheets most commonly contain phthalates, fragrances, MIT, artificial coloring, and also quaternary ammonium compounds (aka quats) that make clothes feel soft and wearable right out of the wash, but some are known to trigger asthma and may be toxic to the reproductive system.[61] Wool balls can serve as dryer sheets to reduce wrinkles, and essential oil can be added for scent if desired.

When considering household products for replacement, consider all of the following:

- Laundry detergent and other laundry products
- Dishwash soap (both for hand washing and machine washing)
- Candles
- Air fresheners
- Cleaning supplies

Fortunately, many brands are now available that utilize non-toxic cleaning agents made from natural products. The following are all brands whose mission is really to create a safer, healthier way to clean, and who are very particular about the ingredients they use:

- Branch Basics
- Better Life
- Meliora
- Greenshield Organics
- Attitude
- Pure Natural
- Truly Free

These products are ideal as they are incredibly clean as well as effective. However, many of these types of products are not always readily available in typical retail settings and require purchasing online or at specialty health stores.

One of the easiest things you can do is screen all of your household products for "fragrance" on the ingredient label to avoid unnecessary phthalate exposure. Unfortunately, many of the products that are on the shelves of natural food stores, like Seventh Generation, Method, and Ecover, contain ingredients like "fragrance," ethoxylated ingredients, and MIT.

Clothing

While clothing is not often considered for its toxicity, the truth is that many of our clothes are created from plastics and synthetic fibers. While you may consider switching some of your clothes to organic fibers, such as cotton, wool, or silk, there are some key pieces of clothing to consider changing.

The rise of athleisure clothing for women has contributed to more women wearing yoga pants and leggings for a variety of different reasons. They're comfortable, they're flattering, and you can easily take clothing from your workout to the grocery store or a coffee shop, and lounge in them at home. But with this rise of athleisure, there's also been an increase in women who wear these types of clothing and the synthetic fibers they often contain directly against their reproductive organs. That's right, I'm talking about not wearing underwear with your yoga pants, and if this is you, you'll want to consider how this might be impacting your toxicity and fertility.

Many yoga pants are made from polyester, nylon, and Lycra, all of which are synthetic materials derived from crude oil that often shed microfibers. Keep in mind that the vaginal epithelium is just like any other skin, and as such, can absorb toxins, but this epithelium is a mucosal membrane, similar to the inside of your mouth or the gut lining, meaning that it's more susceptible to absorbing toxins when in direct contact with synthetic materials. Many of the toxicities seen in clinical practice relate to these types of exposures.

To avoid exposure, you might consider completely changing the materials you wear to include more natural fibers like organic cotton, or at a minimum, wearing organic cotton underwear. Similarly, cotton and wool are the only fabrics that should be worn directly against the skin for underwear, as well as around the breasts.

Unfortunately, not much data currently exists on the impacts of these synthetic fibers for women, since most research is conducted on men across the board. However, polyester has also been shown to impact spermatogenesis for men in several studies.[62][63]

Chapter 10

Addressing Mold Exposures and Mold in Your Body

CORE PRINCIPLE THREE: If you suspect the presence of mycotoxins, assess excretion levels, test your home, and act accordingly.

If you're experiencing symptoms associated with mold toxicity and mycotoxin illness, you'll want to consider testing yourself for the excretion of mycotoxins, first and foremost. Determining what you're excreting and at what levels can be incredibly insightful, not only for beginning to develop a game plan to address these biotoxins that inhibit so many systems in the body related to fertility, but also for ensuring you have a way to monitor progress – with the goal of transferring as few toxins as possible to your future child in utero.

To determine the presence and impact of mycotoxins in your body, urine testing is one of the best ways to measure the active excretion of mycotoxins; such testing can help you tie their presence back to your symptoms and help you determine if an environmental mold should be considered.

While mycotoxin urine testing can help confirm the presence and harm of these biotoxins, it won't tell you if you are currently being exposed. Mycotoxin testing can indicate exposure to molds that have colonized the body (typically the sinuses and GI tract) at any point in your past. For many, this is an exposure that happened in childhood that didn't cause symptoms or illness to occur immediately, but have been low-brewing for years, and often decades, until the immune system is compromised, allowing for the proliferation of mold and thus, an increase in the production of mycotoxins that result in symptoms.

A positive urine test is a crucial component of healing as it helps you better understand impacted detox pathways and binding needs. Not all mycotoxins are bound by the same binders. For instance, while activated charcoal is commonly used as a binder to mop up and pull mycotoxins out of the body, it does not work on all types of mycotoxins. Note that if you have symptoms of mycotoxin illness but do not have mycotoxins present in the urine, this may not necessarily rule out mycotoxins as a contributing factor for you. In fact, detoxification pathways and kidney impairment in particular can occur as a result of long-standing mold illness. This is why tying your symptoms back to lab findings is so crucial.

To help prevent this "false negative" from happening, it's important to provoke excretion with sweating or lymphatic drainage, as discussed in Chapter 8. Mycotoxin excretion can increase by 10-fold, 4–6 hours after a sauna, so you may consider using a sauna nightly for one week and then conduct sample collection to ensure an accurate look at excretion levels. Mycotoxin urine testing always requires that a sample be collected first thing in the morning, when concentrations of toxins in urine are at their highest.

VCS testing

The Visual Contrast Sensitivity test, or VCS, was originally created in the 1940s as a way to detect exposure to bioweapons among soldiers. Adapted to its current form by Ritchie Shoemaker, this test evaluates two sets of nerves in the eye that allow a person to differentiate between white, black, and gray on a gray background. Visual contrast can be depleted in a person who is inflamed or atrophied by mycotoxins because some of the visual center regions become negatively affected.

It has been found that a subject with biotoxin-associated illness will demonstrate a deficit in this non-invasive neurological evaluation, in that they will not be able to identify the direction of various patterns presented. A failed test indicates retinal inflammation, which is often due to mold.

The VCS is an online test that is very low cost and an initial screening tool for mold toxicity. Passing the test does not mean mycotoxins are not an issue, but failing the test is an excellent clue that they are, as around 92% of those affected by mold will fail this test.[1] False positives are quite rare, and it's important to consider that positive results may also be indicative of Lyme disease or mercury toxicity.

This test can be taken at www.vcstest.com.

What to do if you think you are experiencing mycotoxin illness

If you suspect that mold exposure and mycotoxins could be impacting your health, it's important to first consider an exposure timeline.

- Is it possible that there is mold in your current home?
- Does your current home have a history of water damage?
- Is there a point in time that your health significantly decreased or mold symptoms arose? Where were you living at that time?

When in doubt, it's always best to rule out the presence of mold in your current home. It can be an additional step (and investment), but it will help ensure that you are covering all of the bases to promote healing. Not all mold is visible in our homes or creates a "musty" smell, which means you need to explore all options via comprehensive testing.

Consider mold testing in your home

The number-one rule of mold exposure with toxicity is to reduce, if not completely eliminate, mold exposure. For this reason, it's incredibly important to screen your home for mold, at a minimum. While mold can be present in our homes, it can also be present in our workplace, vehicles, and schools. Consider where you spend the most time and where you experience the most symptoms to determine the most influential location for testing, given your circumstances.

There are two tests to consider when testing your environment: the EMMA and the ERMI.

Environmental Mold and Mycotoxin Assessment (EMMA)

This test is conducted by RealTime Laboratories and tests for 10 of the most toxigenic molds associated with their associated 16 mycotoxins. Testing requires a small cutout of an HVAC filter or a swab of dust from an area where you can see mold or suspect it to be present. The kit is packaged with two sterile swabs and a sterile piece of gauze to help you collect a sample. Results are received via email in 7–10 business days and will note levels of both molds and mycotoxins that were screened to determine if there is a harmful toxin that needs remediating in your home. This is our top recommendation for DIY home diagnostic testing, due to the ease of test interpretation and the fact that it measures for both mold and mycotoxins.

Environmental Relative Moldiness Index

The Environmental Relative Moldiness Index (ERMI) is a research tool developed by EPA scientists for estimating mold contamination. It tests for 26 different water damage-associated molds and an additional 9 common indoor molds. In order to use this tool most effectively, the sample needs to be compared to a national database. The basis of this test rests on the findings related to 1,096 homes that were sampled across the U.S. as part of the 2006 American Healthy Home Survey conducted by the Department of U.S. Housing and Urban Development and the EPA. Individual results, ranked from lowest to highest level of "moldiness," were used to create a national Relative Moldiness Index (RMI). When you complete this test, your sample is compared against these rankings to determine danger level.

Unfortunately, while ERMI is one of the most respected mold tests in the U.S., it's not the easiest to interpret on your own, and for that reason I recommend utilizing the EMMA test to determine the presence and severity of mold and mycotoxins in your home.

If you don't find mold or mycotoxins in your environment, then you can safely move forward with your efforts without worrying about any remediation needs.

In the event you do find mold or mycotoxins in your environment, you should consider leaving the environment or implementing proper remediation.

There are several steps required for a comprehensive and effective remediation, which we outline later in this chapter. Finding a reputable remediation company is crucial, and it is often a significant investment to have it done properly.

Remediation will likely require the replacement of the impacted materials, which can include drywall, wood beams, carpet, and more.

A note on "fogging"

I'm often asked about "fogging" for the remediation for mold, as it is a more affordable option that many remediation companies offer, but it is unfortunately not an effective solution.

Fogging is very similar to an aerosol and does not penetrate hard surfaces. The cleaning solution combines with the oxygen in the air to create a vapor that causes droplets to fall on area surfaces and weigh down the mold spores. This process takes several hours to several days, depending on your square footage, and it only works to deactivate and remove mold spores attached to the air particles.

This process latches onto the spores, or microbial Volatile Organic Compounds (VOCs), that the vapor comes in contact with on treated surfaces and works to eliminate the "musty" smell in the air, but it does not actually kill the spores, and more importantly, it does not kill the original source of the mold, which will continue to release spores into the air after the treatment is finished.

Yes, it will smell nicer. Yes, your air will test cleaner. But in a matter of hours or days, your mold problem will return. The problem is that this treatment is not invasive enough and does not affect the underlying surfaces that actually contain the source of your mold. In essence, this is a "band-aid" fix.

While waiting for remediation, if you know there is a moldy area in your home, please follow these instructions:

- If at all possible, do not touch or disturb the mold, as this will release spores into the air that are then available for inhalation and may impact your family's health. Leave the mold removal and cleaning to trained professionals who will have the appropriate safety gear and resources to ensure its removal.
- If you are very sick, it's important to leave the environment, and do not disturb mold at any cost. This means you won't want to touch or brush against visible mold or move any materials that mold is growing on.
- Never use bleach on mold, as this releases mycotoxins that can then be inhaled.
- Any time you are in a contained moldy environment, such as an attic or basement, consider wearing an N95 mask to reduce inhalation of these toxic substances.
- Open windows to allow for air flow and fresh air.
- Consider air purification to filter mycotoxins from the air, as discussed in Chapter 9.

Mycotoxins can live in a variety of different porous surfaces in the home, which is what makes remediation so daunting and exhaustive. Here are a number of other sources of mycotoxins to consider if mold has been confirmed in your home as part of your remediation efforts.

- Books
- Paper
- Upholstery

- Mattresses
- Bedding
- Appliances
- Rugs
- Towels
- Wood
- Leather
- Electronics
- Plastics
- Clothing
- Photos

These items are safe and not impacted by mold spores and mycotoxins:

- Metals
- Ceramics
- Glass
- Clothing
- Artwork (as long as it is not real canvas)

When moving out of a location with mold, taking contaminated personal items, such as furniture and clothing, can continue to cause reactions. Proper cleaning of all personal items when leaving a mold-ridden environment is recommended.

If you find mycotoxins as a result of urine testing, you'll want to take a three-pronged approach to effectively support detoxification.

Step 1: Support natural detoxification efforts

Our bodies are designed to tolerate and withstand exposure to these type of toxins, but sometimes we need a little additional support. This is especially true if you have been impacted by mold due to impacts to the liver and GI tract, which both play a crucial role in the detoxification process to remove these toxins on a daily basis.

You'll want to ensure that you are able to properly eliminate mycotoxins from the body as a first step before moving into the following prongs of support. What we do not eliminate, we recirculate. This means that we need to ensure drainage is supported, as outlined in Chapter 8.

When it comes to mycotoxin illness, we want to consider a few key avenues for support.

Regular bowel elimination

Are you having at least one bowel movement per day? If not, you are recirculating toxins, including mycotoxins, due to not excreting them.

Because of the way that mycotoxins impact the migratory motor complex, constipation is one of the most common symptoms associated with mold toxicity. You'll want to ensure daily bowel movements are happening by supporting elimination.

This type of support can provide short-term, symptomatic relief while the deeper issue of mold toxicity is addressed.

Magnesium oxide has a natural laxative effect because it helps osmotically mediate water retention. It also relaxes the muscles in the digestive tract to help to move stool through the intestines without contributing to the release of water via the bowels, like magnesium citrate can. For this reason, it's often a better choice for constipation symptom relief compared to magnesium citrate, which can contribute to systemic dehydration and worse constipation over time.

Senna tea is another herbal support for the relief of constipation and contains compounds that have a strong laxative effect.[2] They work by irritating the lining of the colon to promote colon contractions and bowel movements, as a result. Senna also prevents water and electrolytes from being reabsorbed from the colon, which increases the amount of fluid in the intestine to soften the stool and can also lead to diarrhea in large doses.[3]

Coffee or water enemas can also provide symptom relief for constipation but are more time-intensive and are best utilized as a back-up option to support bowel movements. Since enemas work by breaking up and loosening impacted stool, they can provide symptom relief but may not support the complete evacuation needed to promote detoxification efforts.

Hydration

As mycotoxins are excreted via the urinary tract, it's important to ensure that proper hydration and electrolytes support is in place. The kidneys are one of our primary detoxification organs and can carry much of the burden when it comes to mycotoxin illness, which is why it's not uncommon to experience urinary tract infections or irritation in the urinary tract during the excretion of mycotoxins.

Refer to our hydration guidelines in Chapter 16 for more information on how much water to drink, ensuring a quality water type, and introducing electrolytes to support detoxification via the kidneys.

Liver detoxification

As one of the primary organs impacted by mycotoxins, the liver often needs additional ongoing support during the process of detoxification from mycotoxins. This can be done in a number of ways, including dietary choices and supplementation, which we'll discuss in depth in Chapter 12, as well as liver detoxification support, including castor oil packs and coffee enemas, as discussed in Chapter 8.

Lymphatic drainage

As we discussed earlier, the lymphatic system plays a crucial role in detoxification by filtering damaged cells and metabolic byproducts via lymph nodes, to be released into the lungs, bowels, and urine for excretion. Stagnation in the lymphatic system can impair progress in mycotoxin removal. Supporting lymph drainage is essential as part of resolving mycotoxin illness. Refer to Chapter 8 for more strategies for supporting this system, with particular attention paid to dry brushing and supporting the six major lymph nodes.

Skin and sweating

Mycotoxins, and many other toxins, are preferentially excreted through the skin and therefore, sweating is an easy way to effectively support their removal. Daily dermal excretion tends to be a primary route for eliminating heavy metals, as they can't pass through the kidney capillaries. Exercise increases the breakdown of fatty acids and mobilizes lipids along with stored mycotoxins from stored body fat. Refer to Chapter 8 for more information on the importance of sweating and strategies to support daily dermal excretion.

Important note: If you are unable to sweat easily, it's important to not force sweating through heat exposure. Difficulty sweating can be a sign of mitochondrial dysfunction or lymphatic stagnation in the skin. Refer to Chapter 11 for more information regarding supporting mitochondria, and prioritize dry brushing of the skin for lymphatic drainage.

Step 2: Bind to mycotoxins

Utilizing binders based on the findings of your mycotoxin testing is crucial to help carry these toxins out of the body effectively, but first it's helpful to understand how binders work. Different mycotoxins are bound and excreted by bound for excretion by different binders. A mold-literate practitioner can assist in selecting the binders that are suited for your mycotoxin burden and tolerated by your body.

Binding agents attach themselves to the circulating toxins and allow them to be properly eliminated. Binders are most effective in the intestinal tract, where they can mop up toxins being released through bile production.[4] Many binders in effect block enterohepatic recirculation. This means that rather than allowing bile to be recycled, the bile and its bound toxins are sequestered and then excreted via bowel movements. As such, binders are aiming to bind both the bile and the toxins.

It's important to note that these binders also bind cholesterol, hormones, minerals, and possibly some fat-soluble nutrients, which is why they are intended for short-term use only.

It's not uncommon for binders to mobilize toxins faster than a compromised detox system can process them, making a mold-toxic person feel worse. For that reason, more is not necessarily better, and increasing your dosage slowly over time may be necessary to avoid symptoms.

If binders make you feel worse, you may need to decrease the dosage or even remove them entirely before starting again slowly to find a tolerable dose. Any increase in symptoms, including nausea, diarrhea, fatigue, sleep disruption, or anything else that crops up suddenly, is a sign to slow down.

Here are some of the most commonly detected mycotoxins and the most effective binders for each of them. [Sources for list: Chapter 10, References 5 to 31]

Activated Carbon: Aflatoxin, Ochratoxin A, Zearalenone, Fumonisins (B1, B2, B3), Patulin, Macrocyclic Trichothecenes, Fusarium Trichothecenes

Activated Charcoal: Aflatoxin, Ochratoxin A, Zearalenone, Fumonisins (B1, B2, B3), Citrine and Dihydrocodeine, Patulin, Mycophenolic Acid, Chaetoglobosin A, Macrocyclic Trichothecenes, Fusarium Trichothecenes

Alfalfa Fiber: Zearalenone, Fusarium Trichothecenes

Beta Glucan: Aflatoxin, Ochratoxin A, Zearalenone, Fumonisins (B1, B2, B3), Patulin, Fusarium, Trichothecenes

Cholestyramine: Ochratoxin A, Fumonisins (B1, B2, B3), Mycophenolic Acid, Chaetoglobosin A, Fusarium Trichothecenes

Chlorella: Aflatoxin, Chaetoglobosin A

Clays: Aflatoxin, Ochratoxin A, Zearalenone, Enniatin B1, Fumonisins (B1, B2, B3), Patulin, Gliotoxin, Mycophenolic Acid, Chaetoglobosin A, Fusarium Trichothecenes

Diatomaceous Earth: Aflatoxin, Ochratoxin A, Zearalenone, Fusarium Trichothecenes

Fulvic Acid: Zearalenone, Fumonisins (B1, B2, B3)

Glucomannan: Aflatoxin, Ochratoxin A, Zearalenone, Fusarium Trichothecenes

Humic Acid: Aflatoxin, Ochratoxin A, Zearalenone, Fumonisins (B1, B2, B3), Fusarium Trichothecenes

NAC: Ochratoxin, Gliotoxin, Chaetoglobosin A, Fusarium Trichothecenes

Probiotics: Aflatoxin, Ochratoxin A, Zearalenone, Fumonisins (B1, B2, B3), Patulin, Trichothecenes, Fusarium Trichothecenes

Spore-Based Probiotics: Aflatoxin, Ochratoxin A, Zearalenone, Enniatin B1, Fumonisins (B1, B2, B3), Citrine and Dihydrocodeine, Patulin, Gliotoxin, Mycophenolic Acid, Chaetoglobosin A, Fusarium Trichothecenes

Zeolites: Aflatoxin, Ochratoxin A, Zearalenone, Fumonisins (B1, B2, B3), Mycophenolic Acid

Step 3: Fight back against proliferation of mycotoxins

The first piece of promoting the removal of mycotoxins is to ensure that you are not inadvertently contributing to the proliferation of mycotoxins in the body through dietary choices.

Carbohydrates, both naturally occurring and processed sugars, contribute to the nourishment of fungal infections. It's important to drastically reduce the consumption of these types of foods, especially table sugar and all other simple, fast-releasing sugars, such as fructose, lactose, maltose, glucose, mannitol, and sorbitol. This includes honey and natural sugar syrup-type products such as maple syrup and molasses. It also includes all candies, sweets, cakes, cookies, and baked goods.

High-sugar containing fruits include pineapple, mango, banana, melons, oranges, and grapes. Low-sugar containing fruits include organic berries, apples, lemons, and limes.

Complete restriction is not the goal here, as carbohydrates are an essential macronutrient for hormone and brain function, but we do want to be mindful of consumption. This is especially true if you have any concerns surrounding blood sugar regulation, which we'll discuss in more depth in Chapter 16.

You may also want to reduce the consumption of mold- and yeast-containing foods, such as cheeses (moldy cheese options, buttermilk, sour cream, and sour milk products), alcoholic drinks (including beer, wine, cider, whiskey, brandy, gin, and rum), processed and smoked meats, fruit juices, and dried fruits.

What about the consumption of edible fungi and medicinal mushrooms?

Based on the concept of "like heals like," I don't find that the removal of edible fungi such as mushrooms and truffles, or the consumption of medicinal mushrooms like reishi, cordyceps, and lion's mane is necessary, as their benefits override any potential harm by consuming fungi during a fungal overgrowth in the body. In fact, these types of mushrooms can be immunomodulating, which can be helpful for those experiencing mold toxicity.[32] It's important to keep in mind that we are all unique and that if you don't respond well to them, removal may be necessary.

Coffee beans are one of the top contenders for food-based mycotoxin exposure. Several studies have found measurable levels of mycotoxins in coffee beans - both roasted and unroasted - as well as brewed coffee. This is true for coffee beans from around the globe, with 33% of green coffee beans from Brazil showing low levels of ochratoxin A[33] and 18% of coffee beans from Portugal containing ochratoxin A.[34] Aflatoxins have been found in green coffee beans, with the highest levels occurring in decaffeinated beans, and research showed that roasting the beans only reduced the levels by 42–55%.[35]

Don't worry; this doesn't mean you have to give up coffee entirely, but you may want to find a mold-free organic coffee option to switch to. There are many brands on the market if you simply search for "mold-free coffee" or switch to an adaptogenic coffee.

Impaired Detox Pathways

Different mycotoxins utilize specific detoxification pathways for excretion, so when you know which mycotoxins are present in your body, you can more effectively support the necessary pathways for excretion. Below are the Phase II liver detoxification pathways impacted by some of the most common mycotoxins.

Acetylation Pathway by: Doxynivalenol, Roridin E

Amino Acid Conjugation by: Ochratoxin A

Glutathione conjugation by: Aflatoxin B1, Ochratoxin A

Glucuronidation by: Alternaniol, Diacetoxyscripenol, Doxynivalenol (DON), Fusarium, Mycophenolic Acid, Nivalenol, Ochratoxin A, Riordin E, Sterigmatocystin, T-2 Toxin, Verrucarin A, Zearalenone

Methylation by: Alternaniol, Fusarium, Zearalenone

Sulfation by: DON (Doxynivalenol), T-2 Toxin

You can find more information on supporting each of these pathways with dietary and supplementation strategies in Chapter 12.

Antifungal agents

Once binders have been established and are well-tolerated, you may consider the introduction of antifungal agents to support the eradication of any mycotoxins present in the body, especially the GI tract.

Because mycotoxins can be incredibly difficult to eradicate in the body, more than one antifungal agent may need to be used at a time, and agents may need to be rotated in order to achieve complete resolution.

Below are some of our preferred antifungal agents for you to consider:

- Caprylic acid
- Monolaurin or Lauricidin
- Pau d'arco
- Olive leaf
- Oregano oil
- Garlic
- Berberine
- Undecylenic acid (Calcium Undecylenate)
- Grape seed extract
- Horopito
- Saccharomyces boulardii
- Aloe vera

Utilize two antifungals for 4 weeks minimum, then rotate to two different antifungals for best results. Resolving mold toxicity and particularly the colonization of mold in the body can take a prolonged period of time. It's often a 6–12 month process alongside balancing other gut imbalances, supporting nutrient depletions, and nourishing organs impacted by mold.

Sinus support

Fungal infections of mold not only colonize the GI tract, but since inhalation is the primary route of exposure, it's not uncommon to see colonization of the sinuses and respiratory tract. This is why respiratory and sinus symptoms are so prevalent for mold toxicity.

By utilizing nasal supports, you'll more effectively support the removal of mycotoxins, regardless of the presentation of sinus symptoms. Keep in mind that mold can proliferate in any spaces that are warm and moist, making your sinus cavity, where the mucous membranes are continuously warm and wet, a perfect environment for proliferation.

Sinus sprays and rinses that include agents such as xylitol, Citricidal, and homeopathic antifungals, such as citrus limona, can be utilized to support this process. To use these sinus sprays effectively, it's important to follow the recommended dosage and use the spray twice daily. After spraying the solution up into the sinuses, turn your head side to side, trying to touch your ear to each shoulder, as well as leaning forward and getting upside down if possible. This ensures the solution reaches into all corners of the sinus cavities, of which there are eight in total.

Mold can be an insidious pathogen that finds refuge in our bodies. While it's important to remove any possible exposure sources, it's not uncommon for mold to be difficult to eradicate despite no longer being exposed. A typical timeline for the eradication of mold and healing of the body in the aftermath is 6–12 months. Your timeline may be longer, but do not fret, as you'll see changes along the way. Mold, however, can be a big root cause of infertility for both men and women.

Re-testing for mycotoxins with a Visual Contrast Sensitivity (VCS) test and urine testing is a great way to ensure you've completed your work, track progress, and have tangible data to put alongside your daily experience.

Note that mycotoxins and fungi in general can be harbored inside other pathogens in the body, such as helminths (parasites), which we'll discuss in depth in Chapter 13. These normal gut pathogens undergo varying life cycles and serve as a protective mechanism for us by harboring mycotoxins to prevent ongoing circulation. As its life cycle ends, a pathogen's body breaks down, and with this comes the release of any of the contents of their body, including mycotoxins. Consider your symptoms to determine if parasitic overgrowths should be part of your healing journey.

Fungal overgrowths can also occur in the presence of metal toxicity. Consider what coinciding toxins may be contributing to a susceptibility for mycotoxin illness.

At some point, you may realize that you've come into contact with mold again. It's easy to feel anxious about mold creating a home inside of you once again, especially after you've gone through so much to rebalance things in the first place.

It's important to understand that mold is natural, and in many cases, unavoidable. We've all checked into a hotel only to find our room is a little musty for our liking, and these are the breeding grounds for mold. When we remove toxicity in our bodies, we're able to build a robust immune system capable of fighting against any pathogens that may come our way.

Chapter 11

Supporting Mitochondrial Function for Healthy Organs

CORE PRINCIPLE FOUR: Support mitochondrial function and energy production in the body.

We all remember having the concept of the "powerhouse of the cell" drilled into our heads in high school, but we likely didn't realize how important mitochondria are to our overall health and our ability to conceive and carry to term.

Keep in mind that we have 30-trillion cells in our body, and each of those cells contains on average, 1,000–10,000 mitochondria. Female egg cells contain the most mitochondrial per cell in the whole body, containing not only 100,000 mitochondria to support the role of fertilization and embryonic development, but also 50,000–150,000 copies of the mitochondrial genome.[1] Our children also inherit mitochondrial DNA exclusively from their mother, so it's crucial that we support healthy function. This is just one more way that we give our offspring everything, so let's give them the best we possibly can.

Mitochondria are membrane-bound cell organelles that live in the nucleus of cells. They generate most of the chemical energy needed to power the cell's biochemical reactions, and damage to mitochondria can then impair the function of organs and our overall energy levels. In other words, our mitochondria fuel cellular function and energy. The energy produced by each mitochondrion is stored in a small molecule called adenosine triphosphate (ATP).

Our mitochondria are also involved with programmed cell death, otherwise known as apoptosis. This is beneficial cell death that occurs as a normal and controlled part of eliminating unwanted cells (such as cells that are virus-infected, cancerous, or old).

In addition to their role as the powerhouse of cells, mitochondria also serve as the "canary in the coal mine" when it comes to the toxicity we face in our lives. They are the first part of the body to be impacted, due to their small size, and this has far reaching implications. Mitochondria are either calm and producing ATP, or in the presence of a stressor, ATP can leave and signal for the immune system. All stressed cells ultimately leak ATP and trigger a cell danger response (CDR).[2]

The first phase of CDR response can result in a number of health conditions where infections are able to overtake cells, including allergies, asthma, skin infections, Candida, parasitic infections, H. pylori and even Lyme disease. As CDR progresses, more serious conditions, such as diabetes, hypertension, heart disease, inflammatory bowel disease (including Crohn's and ulcerative colitis), cirrhosis and cancers have been noted in the literature.[3]

Specifically to hormones, CDR can affect all major endocrine glands. Mitochondria dysfunction and CDR are the major factors in what is commonly referred to as "adrenal fatigue." These mitochondria also play a crucial role in the synthesis of hormones like pregnenolone and therefore, progesterone.[4]

The cell from the ovary that undergoes cell division (known as an oocyte) to create an ovum for fertilization requires certain levels of ATP for the developing embryo until the blastocyst stage of development.[5] There's growing evidence that suggests that embryo potential could be related to the ability of the oocyte mitochondria to generate energy to support cellular division.[6] This means that mitochondria play a critical role in the very initial stages of pregnancy, as well as in carrying to full term.

Furthermore, human fertility and early embryogenesis may be affected by either point mutations or deletions in mitochondrial DNA. Mitochondrial function has even been associated with ovarian aging,[7] with many studies showing that support to optimize mitochondrial function drastically prolongs the age at which women can conceive.

How they are damaged

Damage to mitochondria doesn't just occur naturally. These parts of the cell have been around for 1.45-billion years – they've "seen some stuff." But nothing prepared them to withstand the incredible levels of toxicity they face in our modern worlds. And while the mitochondria are designed to withstand CDR, and this is a natural and necessary process in the health of cells, the problem comes when cells get stuck in the CDR and are unable to produce adequate ATP to upkeep the health of the cell.

Volatile Organic Compounds (VOCs) damage the membranes of mitochondria, making it more likely that ATP can leave the cell even if not intended to.[8]

Heavy metals wreak havoc on our mitochondria and impact their ability to produce energy. They disrupt cellular events, including growth, proliferation, differentiation, damage-repairing processes, and apoptosis.[9] Arsenic, aluminum, and thallium in particular also disrupt enzymes that transport nutrients into the mitochondria.[10] Lead has the capacity to completely choke off the mitochondria.[11] [12]

Many mycotoxins target mitochondria, causing damage and reduced ATP production.[13]

Glyphosate-based herbicides can also modify mitochondrial membranes. Alterations in the mitochondrial bioenergetic reactivity as a result of glyphosate have drastic consequences for cellular function by changing the bioenergetic charge and balance of the cell.[14] More specifically, glyphosate impacts the mitochondrial function of sperm and impairs their fertilization capacity.

Another consequence of high toxin burden is that the mitochondria react by decreasing their oxygen consumption. This raises the oxygen concentration within the mitochondria itself, increasing a process known as cellular redox, which is when cells increase oxidation in order to shield themselves from further injury.[15] This drop in oxygen consumption means the mitochondria can no longer fuel cellular respiration, resulting in extreme fatigue.[16]

Lack of sleep can also contribute to mitochondrial dysfunction. In 2018, a study using a combination of in-vitro and in-vivo models of human skin fibroblasts and mice established a link between sleep rhythms and mitochondrial health.[17] Analysis showed that even short-term sleep deprivation affects mitochondrial bioenergetic capacity.[18]

Furthermore, chronic stress exposure can lead to molecular and functional recalibrations among mitochondria.[19]

Lack of exercise can contribute to poor mitochondrial function, while excess exercise can also deplete mitochondria. It's a "goldilocks situation" where we need just the right amount of exercise to support the health of our mitochondria. Research on mitochondria in skeletal muscle shows that exercise can produce an increase in mitochondria by up to 40%.[20]

The key with exercise is to recognize when it's supportive, and when it's acting as just another stressor on the body. Doing difficult workouts every day without rest in between is just as damaging to your mitochondria as any other toxin. But done properly and with plenty of rest, strengthening your muscles with weight training can help increase mitochondria production and efficiency over time.

When you combine our overall toxin burden impacting our energy production capacity with the resulting dysfunction throughout the body, and layer on huge amounts of emotional stress, you have a recipe for mitochondrial dysfunction.

How to support mitochondrial function

First and foremost, adequate calorie needs play a role in mitochondrial function. Research shows that calorie restriction and intermittent fasting can reduce mitochondrial biogenesis and function and stimulate mitochondrial death.[21] We'll discuss caloric recommendations more in Chapter 16, but low calorie diets, calorie restriction, and being in a chronic deficit not only impact mitochondrial function systemically but can negatively impact the health of eggs.

Mitochondria are the generators of power in the cell, but also throughout the body. While the thyroid and its associated hormones are responsible for the generation and maintenance of our metabolism, this gland is particularly responsive to other inputs, such as mitochondrial output and adrenal function.[22] As we'll soon discuss, the thyroid plays a critical role in fertilization and early pregnancy and is often a contributing factor to miscarriages or the inability to carry to term, but this process begins in the mitochondria. Without adequate caloric intake (energy through nourishment), mitochondria are unable to support metabolic output needs in the thyroid.

Healthy fat intake is especially important to maintain the mitochondrial membrane, which is primarily composed of the phospholipids. Make no mistake, the superheated, rancid oils such as vegetable and canola oil are inflammatory and destructive to your mitochondria. Omega-3 fatty acids are a critical component for all cell membrane fluidity, intercellular signaling, immune modulation, inflammation, and mitochondrial function. A minimum of 1,000 mg of omega-3 fatty acids, specifically EPA and DHA, is recommended daily to support mitochondrial function, though many need higher doses due to deficiencies, as we'll discuss in more detail in Chapter 15.

You may have heard that CoQ10 is good for egg health, and while this is true, the details of how it supports fertility run much deeper. It plays a key role in the synthesis of ATP. Ubiquinol is the activated form of CoQ10 and especially important for those with high levels of oxidative stress and toxin burden. CoQ10 carries the high-energy electrons through the electron transport train, so deficiency means not only decreased ATP production but also increased electron loss, causing oxidative damage. CoQ10 is also an important intramitochondrial antioxidant.[23] Around 200 mg three times per day is recommended to support mitochondrial function evenly throughout the day.

Foods rich in CoQ10 include organ meats (especially liver and kidney), fatty fish, animal meats, spinach, broccoli, cauliflower, strawberries, oranges, lentils, peanuts, pistachios, and sesame seeds.

Acetyl-l-carnitine

Acetyl-l-carnitine provides carnitine to transport long-chain fatty acids into the mitochondria for energy. Combining acetyl-l-carnitine with alpha lipoic acid has been shown to increase mitochondrial ATP production.[24]

Resveratrol

Resveratrol is a naturally-derived polyphenol antioxidant that protects mitochondria. Resveratrol increases mitochondrial ATP production and protects from the reactive oxygen species (ROS) produced by all mammalian cells that can contribute to mitochondrial damage.[25] Human studies are now showing improved mitochondrial function at surprisingly reasonable dosages, 150 mg four times daily.[26]

Foods rich in resveratrol include peanuts, pistachios, grapes, red and white wine, blueberries, cranberries, and even cocoa and dark chocolate.

N-acetyl-cystine (NAC)

The key role of NAC is to increase intracellular glutathione, which is then pumped into the mitochondria. This glutathione is critical for protection of mitochondria from oxidative damage. Recommended dosage is 500 mg twice daily.

B vitamins are needed to fuel the production of ATP by mitochondria, while optimum serum levels of magnesium are associated with healthy mitochondrial metabolism and nutrient transport. We discuss both of these concepts in depth in Chapter 15. Both of these nutrients are often depleted rapidly when we are exposed to oxidative stress, which we are all chronically exposed to.

Is taking all of these nutrients necessary for supporting healthy mitochondrial function? Absolutely not, but you might experiment with different supports to see how you feel, especially if you suffer from significant fatigue. If you're struggling with energy production at a cellular level, you'll feel it in your daily life. You'll notice how your energy levels increase as your cells are able to function more optimally and nourish themselves.

Lifestyle supports

Your exercise efforts can also promote the health of mitochondria, as increasing muscle mass in particular improves their ability to function at optimal levels.[27] Ultimately, promoting the accumulation and maintenance of lean muscle mass can help support mitochondrial function, which can be acquired through resistance and strength training. Furthermore, long-duration cardio exercises, such as running, biking, and anything that keeps your heart rate up for longer than 45 minutes, can become catabolic, breaking down muscle mass.

Chapter 12
The Pillar of Liver Detoxification

CORE PRINCIPLE FIVE: Support natural detoxification pathways and address dysfunction in the liver.

When you think of the liver, are you mostly thinking about the times you've had a little too much to drink and felt it the next day?

While the liver is important for the detoxification of toxins, like alcohol, its role is much more complex, and alcohol is just one of many toxins that burden our livers. It's also one of the most common areas of dysfunction due to the toxic world we are living in.

The liver is responsible for multiple functions in the body, including the production of bile to assist in the breakdown and absorption of fatty acids, as well as the conjugation of toxins from the body, the storage and metabolism of fat-soluble vitamins, and most importantly, the detoxification of both endogenous and exogenous toxins in the body.[1] It's for this reason that we cannot live without a liver. Without this organ, toxin buildup and recirculation would be far too damaging to the health of all tissues and organs to sustain life.

Though the kidneys play a role in detoxification efforts, this job primarily falls on the liver, which takes both endogenous waste products (such as excess hormones, vitamins, and inflammatory toxins) as well as exogenous toxins (such as heavy metals, chemicals, and medications) and eliminates them from the body.

Detoxification, also known as biotransformation, refers to all the steps involved in the chemical alteration and excretion of both endogenous and exogenous substances. While we are exposed to toxins through the diet, lungs, and skin, not all compounds can be excreted right away. Water-soluble compounds that enter the body can be directly excreted, but fat-soluble compounds must undergo biotransformation for excretion via the bowels.

Here are the three primary phases of detoxification that happen in the liver:

Figure 12.1

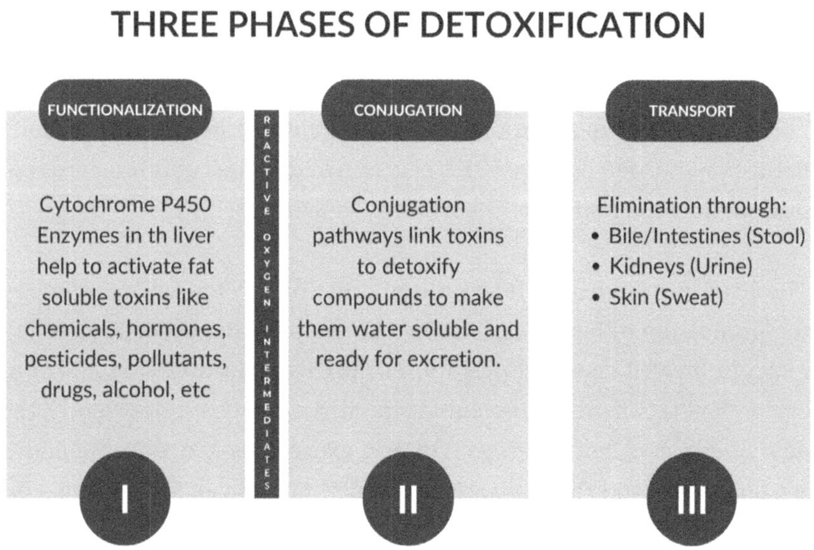

Figure 12.2

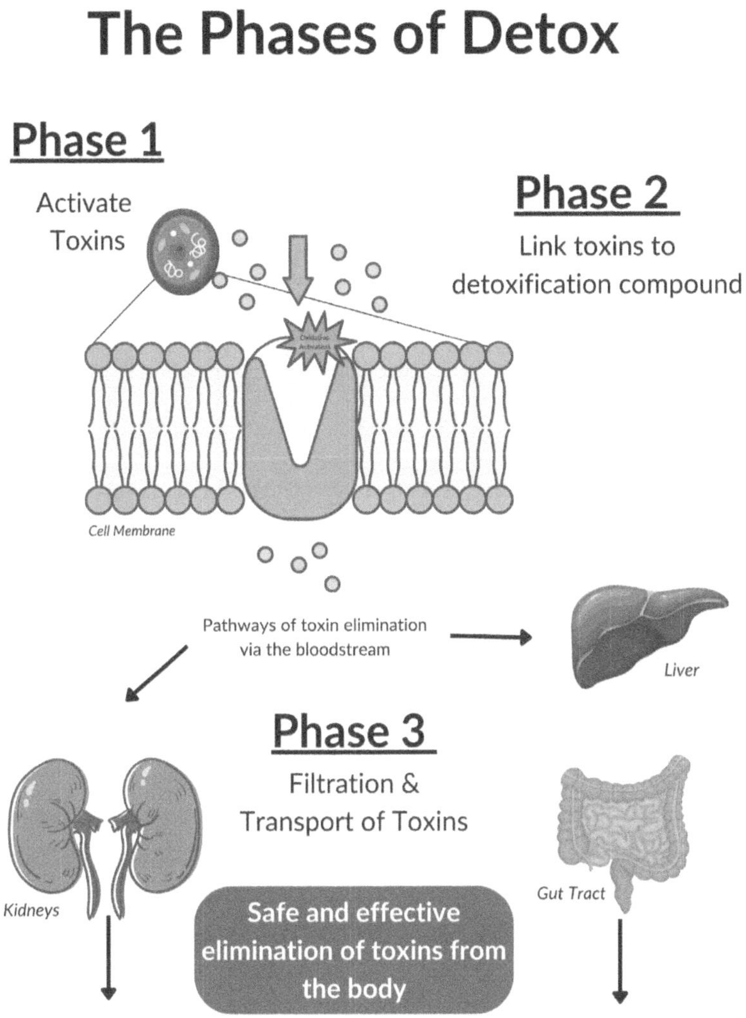

The Phases of Detox
Phase 1
Activate
Toxins
Phase 2
Link toxins to
detoxification compound
Cell Membrane
Pathways of toxin elimination
via the bloodstream
Liver
Phase 3
Filtration &
Transport of Toxins
Kidneys
Gut Tract
Safe and effective
elimination of toxins from
the body

Phase I detoxification

The initial phase is described as functionalization, which involves adding a reactive site on the toxic compound to make it more water-soluble. Toxins must be water-soluble in order to be eliminated effectively. While toxins in this form are water-soluble, they can still be toxic and cause cellular damage.

There are three types of reactions that make up Phase I:

- Oxidation is when an electron is lost, and this is the most common reaction.
- Reduction is when an electron is added.
- Hydrolysis is when a reaction with water breaks a bond to result in two compounds.

The cytochrome P450 (CYP450) enzymes in the liver are responsible for adding the reactive groups via different enzymatic reactions in both oxidation and reduction. The toxic compounds are then converted into intermediary metabolites and the by-product of these reactions are reactive oxygen species. This means that in the process of removing toxins, they become even more toxic and can create oxidative stress in the process.

Remember that glyphosate is known to inhibit CYP450 enzymes,[2] which means that when we are being exposed to glyphosate at even low dosages, especially continuously, this phase of liver detoxification is being impaired. This leads to further toxicity, as the liver is unable to function properly in this first crucial step of the removal of toxins, thus leading to increased toxicity in the body as a whole.

It's also important to note that CYP450 is a heme-based molecule, meaning that adequate iron levels are critical for its formation. Those with insufficient iron intake, absorption, or other factors related to iron anemia may need to promote iron absorption in order to support the robust function of this phase of detoxification. Ensuring adequate chemical digestion and removing chronic gut infections are crucial for ensuring healthy iron levels. We'll discuss more strategies for this in the next chapter on digestion, as well as in Chapter 15.

Among other enzymes, CYP450 enzymes are responsible for drug and hormone breakdown, fatty acid metabolism, bile acid synthesis, vitamin D degradation, cholesterol synthesis, and steroid hormone synthesis. As such, ensuring proper Phase I function is an indirectly crucial component of many factors affecting fertility.

After going through Phase I, a toxin becomes an intermediate metabolite and can then be bound or conjugated in Phase II to prepare them for excretion.

Phase II detoxification

The second phase of detoxification is described as conjugation, which includes adding a water-soluble group to the formed reactive site through a number of different reactions. The goal of this step is to increase the water-solubility of the toxic metabolite, therefore increasing its ability to be eliminated from the body.

Phase II reactions:

- Glucuronidation
- Methylation
- Acetylation
- Glutathione conjugation
- Sulfation
- Amino acid conjugation

Of the various types of conjugation that occur in Phase II detoxification, the following are most relevant to hormone metabolism and therefore, fertility.

Glucuronidation

Glucuronidation makes up 40–70% of Phase II reactions[3] and is critical for the clearance of steroid hormones, such as estrogen, as well as xenobiotics, bilirubin, bile acids, and fat-soluble vitamins. It's also the main pathway for the clearance of mycotoxins.

Glucuronidation utilizes glucuronosyl transferase enzymes, which are synthesized from glucose. This means that healthy blood sugar regulation is a crucial starting point for supporting these pathways, a topic we'll discuss in more depth in Chapter 16.

This conjugation reaction can be undone by elevated levels of beta-glucuronidase enzyme production in the liver, which may be affected by the condition of the intestines. If the intestines have an abundance of abnormal bacteria, the amount of beta-glucuronidase enzyme produced by these bacteria may de-conjugate toxins, including estrogen, which contribute to the recirculation of estrogen and a state of estrogen dominance.

Nutrients to support glucuronidation include cruciferous vegetables, resveratrol, citrus, dandelion, rooibos, honeybush, rosemary, curcumin, astaxanthin, cranberry, echinacea, gingko, green tea, milk thistle, St John's Wort, and valerian.

Methylation

Methylation, also known as methyl metabolism, is the process in which methyl groups are passed from one molecule to another. This process is critical to hundreds of biochemical reactions in the body, and is key to the clearance of heavy metals. Methylation is also used in a wide range of processes throughout the body, including the repair of damaged DNA, the conversion of serotonin to melatonin, the creation of glutathione, and the clearance of histamines.

In order for the liver to have a good supply of methyl groups available, adequate amounts of vitamins B6, B12, and folate are necessary.

Nutrients to support methylation include B12, folate, B6, magnesium, betaine, methionine, cysteine, taurine, DHA, zinc, potassium, riboflavin, niacin, pyridoxine, choline, and sulfur.[4]

Of note, methylation can be impacted by MTHFR genetic mutations. MTHFR is a gene that makes an enzyme called methylenetetrahydrofolate reductase, which is responsible for reducing the buildup of homocysteine in the bloodstream. High levels of homocysteine can lead to inflammation, heart disease, and a wide range of symptoms associated with the deficiency of folate.

These variations in genetics are not as "mutant" as they might seem, with current research estimating that 40% of the population in the United States have one genetic MTHFR variation impacting their ability to undergo the methylation process.[5] Research estimates that those of us with MTHFR changes produce up to 70% less methylfolate than those without the mutation.[6]

There are two presentations of MTHFR mutation: you may be heterozygous, meaning you have one mutation, or homozygous, meaning you have two mutations. Homozygous mutations are more severe and will cause more problems with methylation, but heterozygous mutations can also be problematic, due to bioindividuality – individual variations in nutrition requirements and cross-reacting genetics related to single nucleotide polymorphisms (SNPs).

There are two main types of genetic MTHFR mutations:

- C677T Mutation: Alterations in this gene can lead to high levels of inflammatory homocysteine, which can be measured by blood serum and is linked to heart disease and autoimmune conditions.
- A1298C Mutation: This mutation commonly contributes to mood disorders, as it plays a vital role in neurotransmitter function.

Sulfation

Sulfation is the process by which sulfur groups are added to metabolites to prepare them for easy excretion. Sulfation is important in the clearance of xenobiotics, as well as prescription medications, Tylenol, bile acids, T4, steroids, catecholamines, vitamin D, and cholecystokinin.

To support this process, adequate amounts of foods containing sulfur can be included in the diet, including egg yolks, garlic, onions, and brussels sprouts. Animal protein is another important source of sulfur.

Glutathione conjugation

Glutathione conjugation is the process by which glutathione, another sulfur-containing molecule, is added to metabolized hormones for easy excretion. Glutathione conjugation is used in the Phase II clearance of such substances as prescription medications, Tylenol, heavy metals, petroleum, aflatoxins and other mycotoxins, lipopolysaccharides, and prostaglandins.[7]

Foods such as avocado, walnuts, and asparagus are rich in glutathione, although for many people, food sources alone don't provide enough glutathione to maintain healthy detoxification pathways. Sufficient vitamin C is also important as it stimulates the production of glutathione in the body.

The nutrients that support glutathione conjugation are cruciferous vegetables, alliums, resveratrol, citrus, curcumin, rooibos, honeybush, and liposomal glutathione.

Phase III detoxification

The last phase is focused on excretion, which is the actual removal of toxins from the body. Through Phase I and Phase II detoxification, 80% of toxins are pushed in the bile ducts for elimination,[8] but toxins can also be excreted through urine and the skin.

Transformed substances from Phase II are moved out of the cell into tubules that lead to excretion pathways. Notably, this process is very dependent on magnesium status (e.g., magnesium deficiency impairs the ability of all Phase II detoxification).[9]

Most commonly, the conjugated toxin will then bind with bile and dump via the bile duct into the GI tract for elimination, but it can also be excreted via the hepatic vein to the kidneys, to be eliminated in urine or sweat.[10]

This final phase can be the limiting factor for your ability to remove toxins effectively, based on bile flow. Decreased bile flow (also known as cholestasis) leads to biliary sludge and abnormal bile circulation. When this happens, toxins, pathogenic invaders, and other debris build up in the body, leading to chronic illness and disease. Poor phase III detoxification and low bile flow can also contribute to estrogen dominance, as bile is required for the removal of estrogens.

This phase is particularly important for anyone without a gallbladder or who experiences gallbladder issues, as these can contribute to poor bile flow and therefore inhibit Phase III detoxification. While the liver is responsible for the production of bile, remember that the gallbladder is important for the release of bile into the small intestine to assist in the breakdown of fat-dense foods.

How to know if your liver needs support

Signs of liver toxicity:

- Fatigue[11]
- Brain fog[12]
- Headaches
- Hypersensitivity to chemicals and smells[13]
- Easily intoxicated by alcohol
- Intolerance to fatty foods[14]

- Varicose veins and hemorrhoids [15,16]
- Rectal itching
- Lipomas[17]
- Fatty tumors
- Anger and irritability[18]
- Elevated estrogen levels (and estrogen dominance, including PMS, heavy bleeding, painful periods, clotting)[19]
- Rosacea or flushed face[20]
- Depression
- Excess sweating
- Cellulite[21]
- Red palms and soles of feet
- Rashes of the skin
- High or low blood pressure[22]
- Elevated ALT (above 19 µ/L) and AST (above 21 µ/L) in bloodwork
- Imbalances in the lipid panel (such as low HDL, elevated LDL, elevated cholesterol)

How to support detoxification phases

In addition to choosing organic, non-GMO food to minimize exposure to environmental toxins, you can focus on consuming a robust amount of antioxidant-rich foods to offset reactive oxygen species formed during Phase 1 detoxification. One easy way to do this is to emphasize colorful foods to increase antioxidants, phytonutrient compounds, and diversity in the diet. This helps ensure that the toxic effects of the compounds are minimized while they undergo this process.

You can also focus on nutrients important for multiple Phase II detoxification pathways, such as amino-acid rich foods for amino acid conjugation, glucaric acid-rich foods for glucuronidation, sulfur-rich foods for sulfation, glutathione-rich foods for glutathione conjugation, and foods high in methyl groups for methylation.

Certain types of foods can help facilitate excretion, act as another component of healthy liver detoxification, and support the elimination of toxins through liver, bile, and intestines. Cholagogue foods stimulate the production and release of bile from the liver and gallbladder. This refreshes and cleanses these organs, as well as increases bile in the small intestines.[23] Anything bitter, sour, or oily has a cholagogue effect, but some common cholagogues include:

- Beets
- Dandelion
- Lemons
- Vinegar (such as apple cider vinegar)
- Globe artichoke
- Milk thistle

Fiber is also essential for the elimination of toxins. Dietary fiber has been shown to increase the activity of antioxidant and detox enzymes in your liver, as well as nourish the microbes in the GI tract responsible for secondary bile production.[24] The fiber found in raw carrots is one that deserves special attention, as it binds excess endotoxins and estrogen for elimination from the body.

Raw Carrot Salad Recipe

2 large carrots shredded lengthwise
1 tsp apple cider vinegar
1 tsp coconut oil or extra virgin olive oil
Sea salt (to taste)

In addition to consuming nutrient-rich foods to support detoxification, it's essential to avoid foods that trigger an immune response. Consider food sensitivity testing to identify reactive foods and avoid the foods that typically result in you not feeling your best.

For most people, the elimination of dairy, gluten, and high mercury-containing seafood helps support detoxification efforts, in addition to reducing overall toxin burden through the personal care and home considerations discussed in Chapter 9.

Figure 12.3 FOODS FOR DETOX TABLE

Dairy Alternatives

_________ Servings per day

Low glycemic: Choose unsweetened, limit to 1-2 servings per day (remove if sensitive to dairy)

Meat & Eggs:

"Milk": Almond, coconut, cashews, flax, hemp hazelnut, oat, soy	6-8oz
Kefir (dairy free, active cultures) ●	4-6oz
Yogurt (dairy free) ●	4-6oz
Vegan cheese	1oz

1 serving as listed = 1oz = 25-120kcal, 1-2g protein, 1-4g carbs (Nutritional values vary)

Discuss servings with your provider

Vegetables (Starchy)

_________ Servings per day

Acorn squash	1c
Butternut squash	1c
Parsnips	1/2c
Potato (white, purple ▲)	1/2c
Pumpkin	1/2c
Rutabaga	1/2c
Sweet potato	1/2c
Yam	1/2c

1 serving as listed = 80kcal, 15g carbs (Nutritional values vary)

KEY

MOST DETOXIFYING FOODS (Phase 1 & Phase 2 Inducers)

▲ Phase 2 conjugation inducers

● Phase 3 excretion support

Vegetables (Non-Starchy)

_________ Servings per day

Choose a variety of colorful produce. Focus on cruciferous vegetables and dark leafy greens

Artichokes ▲●
Asparagus ▲
Beets ●
Bok Choy ▲
Broccoli ▲
Brussels sprouts ▲
Cabbage (green, red) ▲
Carrots ▲
Cauliflower ▲
Celery ▲●
Cucumbers ▲
Eggplant
Garlic ▲●
Ginger ▲●
Green beans ▲
Green onion/Scallions ▲
Greens:
Arugula ▲●, Beet, Chard ●, Collard ▲,
Dandelion ▲●, Endive, Kale ▲●,
Microgreens, Mustard ▲●,
Swiss chard, Watercres
Jerusalem artichokes (sunchokes)
Jicama
Leeks ▲
Lettuce ▲
Mushrooms
Onion ▲
Okra ●
Peppers, all ▲
Radishes ▲
Scallions
Sea vegetables
Shallots ▲
Spinach ▲
Sprouts, all
Squash: *Delicata, spaghetti, yellow, zucchini, etc*
Tomato ▲

1 serving = 1/2c cooked, 1c raw = 25kcal, 5g carbs

Fruits

_________ Servings per day

Choose a variety of color to increase antioxidants

Apple ▲●	1 sm
Apricots ▲	4
Banana	1/2 med
Blackberries ▲	3/4c
Blueberries ▲	3/4c
Cherries ▲	12
Cranberries	3/4c
Date	1
Dragon fruit	3/4c
Figs	3
Grapes ▲	15
Grapefruit ▲	1/2 med
Kiwi	1 med
Lemon ▲	1
Lime ▲	1
Mandarin ▲	1
Mango	1/2 sm
Melon, all	1c
Orange ▲	1 med
Papaya	1 c
Peach ▲	1 sm
Pear	1 sm
Pineapple	3/4c
Plantain	1/2 med
Plums ▲	2 sm
Pomegranate seeds ▲	1/2c
Prunes	3 med
Raspberries ▲	1c
Strawberries ▲	1 1/4c

1 serving as listed = 60kcal, 15g carbs

Legumes

_________ Servings per day

Beans: Black beans, Black-eye peas, Broad beans, Chickpeas, Kidney beans, Mung beans ▲, Navy beans, Pinto beans	1/2 c
Green peas ▲	1/2 c
Hummus	1/4 c
Lentils ▲	1/2 c
Peanuts	10
Soybeans: ▲	1/4 c
Edamame ▲	1/4 c
Natto ▲	1 oz
Tofu ▲	2-3 oz
Tempeh ▲	1 oz

1 serving = 110kcal, 15 carbs, 7g protein (Nutritional values vary)

Protein

_________ Servings per day

Organic, grass-fed/pasture raised animals, wild-caught seafood preferred, only low mercury (< 2ppm)

Meat & Eggs: ▲
Beef, Bison, Chicken, Duck, Eggs, Lamb, Pork Rabbit, Turkey, Venison

Fish: ▲
Alaskan pollock, Anchovy, Carp, Cod, Flounder, Mackerel, Perch, Salmon, Sardines, Sea bass, Sole, Trout

Shellfish: ▲
Crab, Lobster, Shrimp, Crayfish, etc.

Mollusks: ▲
Blue mussel, Clam, Oyster, Octopus, Pacific squid, Scallops, Squid, etc.

Protein powders: ▲
Collagen peptides, Whey protein

1 serving = 1oz = 35-75kcal, 5-7g protein, 0-4g fat (Nutritional values vary)

Grains (GF Grains & Alternatives)

_________ Servings per day

Organic, grass-fed/pasture raised animals, wild caught seafood preferred, only low mercury (< 2ppm)

Gluten free grains & Starches:

Amaranth	3/4 c
Bread (GF)	1 slice
Buckwheat/kasha	1/2 c
Cassava	1/2 c
Crackers (GF)	5-10
Corn	1/2 c
Millet	1/2 c
Oats: Rolled, steel-cut, GF ▲	1/2 c
Pasta (GF)	1/2 c
Quinoa	1/2 c
Rice	1/2 c
Sorghum	1/2 c
Tapioca	1/2 c
Taro root	1/2 c
Tiget nut	1/2 c
Teff	3/4 c
Wild rice	1/2 c

1 serving as listed = 80kcal, 15g carbs (Nutritional values vary)

Nuts

_________ Servings per day

Unsweetend recommended

Almonds ▲	6
Brazil Nuts ▲	2
Cashews	6
Hazelnuts	5
Macadamias	2-3
Pecan halves	4
Pine nuts	1T
Pistachios	16
Poppy seeds	2T
Sweet Chestnut	10
Walnut halves ▲	4

1 serving as listed = 45kcal, 5g fat (Nutritional values vary)

Seeds

_________ Servings per day

Unsweetend recommended

Chia seeds ▲●	1T
Flaxseed ▲●	2 T
Hemp seeds ▲	1T
Pumpkin seeds	1 T
Sesame seeds ▲	1 T
Sunflower seeds	1 T

1 serving as listed = 45kcal, 5g fat (Nutritional values vary)

KEY

MOST DETOXIFYING FOODS (Phase 1 & Phase 2 Inducers)

▲ Phase 2 conjugation inducers

● Phase 3 excretion support

Fats & Oils

_________ Servings per day

Choose cold pressed and minimally refined

Fats: ●	2T or 1/8 whole
Avocado	1t - 2T
Coconut (milk, meat, butter)	8
Olives: Black, green, kalamata ▲	1t
Pesto (DF, olive oil)	

Oils: ●	1t

Almond, Avocado, Coconut, Flaxseed
Ghee/clarified butter▲, Hempseed,
Olive (extra virgin), Sesame Oils, Walnut

1 serving as listed ≈ 45cal, 5g fat

Spices

Anise
Basil
Bay leaf
Black pepper
Caraway ▲
Cardamom
Cayenne pepper
Cilantro ●
Cinnamon ●
Clove
Coriander
Cumin ●
Curry powder ▲
Dill ▲
Habanero pepper
Horseradish ▲
Hot paprika pepper
Jalapeno pepper
Lemongrass
Mint ●
Mustard ▲
Nutmeg
Oregano
Parsley
Rosemary
Sage
Thyme
Turmeric
Vanilla bean
Woo-hsiang powder

Miscellaneous

Condiments:
Mustard, Tamari, Coconut aminos, Vinegars, Ketchup

Fermented foods:
Kimchi ●▲, Sauerkraut ●▲

Other:
Aloe vera●, Carob, Cocoa (70% or higher),
Chlorella●, Honey, Maple syrup, Psyllium●

Beverages

Unsweetened preferred

Broth (organic)▲: Bone, meat, vegetable
Coconut water
Coconut water kefir
Filtered water
Kombucha
Sparkling/mineral water
Tea: Black, green▲, oolong, rooibos▲, herbal
Vegetable juice (raw, cold-pressed, green juice)

KEY

MOST DETOXIFYING FOODS (Phase 1 & Phase 2 Inducers)

▲ Phase 2 conjugation inducers

● Phase 3 excretion support

Chapter 13
Restoring Gut Harmony

CORE PRINCIPLE SIX: Restore imbalances in the gut to take the burden off the immune system and endocrine function as a whole.

Imbalances in the gut microbiome, also known as dysbiosis, are one of the leading stressors on women's bodies, as a whole. We have as many bacterial microbes in our gut as there are cells in our entire body – around 38-trillion.[1] When the good bacteria are overrun by harmful, pathogenic organisms, this creates inflammation in the GI tract, impairs chemical digestion and nutrient absorption, and can negatively impact the endocrine system by placing stress on the adrenal glands.

While there is a tiered set of imbalances, these issues do not arise overnight. Many women have life-long gut issues that began when they were children and have never resolved, while others notice a drastic shift that happens at a certain point in their recent past.

Here are some symptoms associated with impaired digestive capacity and microbiome imbalances:

- Belching or gas within an hour of eating
- Heartburn or acid reflux
- Bloating
- Stomach upset by taking vitamins
- Sense of excess fullness after meals
- Feel better skipping breakfast
- Fingernails chip, peel or easily break
- Stomach pains or cramps
- Diarrhea
- Black or tarry-colored stools

- Undigested food in the stool
- Stomach upset by greasy foods
- Fatty or shiny stools
- Nausea
- Light or clay-colored stools
- Hemorrhoids, anal fissures, or varicose veins
- Food allergies
- Pulse elevated after eating
- Hives
- Sinus congestion or having a "stuffy head"
- Alternating from constipation to diarrhea
- Rectal, anal itching
- White-coated tongue
- History of yeast or fungal infections
- Ringworm or nail fungus
- Constipation or difficult-to-pass stool
- Less than 1 bowel movement per day
- Blood in the stool
- Mucus in the stool
- Excess, foul-smelling gas
- Dark circles under your eyes
- Skin issues (rashes, itchy, hives, eczema, or acne)
- Bowel urgency or occasional accidents
- Grinding teeth when asleep
- Hyperactivity tendency (nervousness)
- Anxiety and mood disorders
- Night sweats (not menopausal)
- Anemia (low iron and/or hemoglobin levels on blood test)
- Inability to gain healthy weight
- Unexpected changes in appetite
- Sugar and sweet cravings
- Sore throat (chronic)

While some of these may not appear to relate directly to the digestive system, they shows signs of immune dysfunction as a whole. Since we know that the majority of the immune system resides in the gastrointestinal tract, these are important clues to the presence of dysbiosis. We'll break these symptoms down into specific pathogens in the coming sections.

The colon is also one of our primary drainage pathways. The removal of excrement via the stools is the primary path for toxins to be removed. When this isn't happening routinely, toxins are reabsorbed in the large intestine and begin to recirculate through the body. In other words, if you aren't having at least one bowel movement per day, you're constipated, and you're creating an overly toxic environment.

Phase one: Beneficial bacteria insufficiency

Beneficial bacteria are the cornerstone of microbiome health. We get everything from our mothers - their looks, their genetics, and even their microbiome. Each person's unique microbiome is acquired first in utero, and then through the process of birth. Those born vaginally are exposed to the beneficial bacteria present throughout the vaginal canal, while those born via C-section are born into a sterile environment and exposed to a different set of microbes. We are also inoculated with bacteria through skin-to-skin contact, breastfeeding, and the organisms within our homes as babies. Throughout childhood, we are exposed to a wide range of organisms as we touch everything, place it in our mouths, and begin to build our immune system.

It's estimated that 70–80% of the immune system resides in the intestinal tract.[2] When imbalance in the microbiome exists, immune function can become compromised. In some cases, the immune system upregulates in order to fight off pathogens in the gut, but over time, the immune system can deteriorate as it begins to "lose the war" against pathogens and becomes depleted and unable to keep up with demands.

Outside of immune function, beneficial bacteria are also responsible for the development of neurotransmitters, and 95% of the body's serotonin, our "happy hormone," is produced in the digestive tract,[3] meaning that the microbiome plays an integral role in mental health as well.

Beneficial bacteria also play a role in the production of enzymes important for the metabolism of carbohydrates, proteins, plant polyphenols, and vitamins.[4] These beneficial bacteria also produce vitamins that are then absorbed in the colon, such as vitamin K. This is particularly important as daily intake of vitamin K is often insufficient to support systemic needs, and it also plays an important role in blood clotting and therefore, is protective against miscarriage.[5]

The microbiome of the gut influences many other microbiomes of the body, including the skin, sinuses, reproductive organs, and urinary tract.[6 7 8]

Insufficiency of these bacteria can contribute to overgrowths of other organisms that normally reside in the gut, such as yeast and parasites. One of the primary roles of beneficial bacteria is to crowd out the presence of these microbes, but when beneficial bacterial levels drop, it creates an opportunity for these opportunists to proliferate and create inflammation. Antibiotic use (and overuse) also commonly contribute to yeast overgrowths, as they not only damage harmful bacteria when they are used, but also negatively impact beneficial bacteria. As a result, use of antibiotics can be even more inflammatory and upregulate the immune system; importantly, a calm immune system is crucial for implantation and the ability to sustain a pregnancy.

So what causes an insufficiency of beneficial bacteria in the first place?

Antibiotic overuse is one of the leading contributing factors for insufficient beneficial bacteria levels, as antibiotics are used to eradicate harmful bacterial infections, but also damage the integrity of beneficial bacteria in the process. In 2021 alone, 221-million antibiotics were prescribed, the equivalent of 636 antibiotics prescriptions per 1,000 people.[9] This doesn't take into account the 32% of births that occur via C-section,[10] where antibiotics administered to the mother during delivery are then passed to children via the bloodstream and breastmilk. Two-thirds of children also receive at least one course of antibiotics by the time they turn one year old.[11]

Poor dietary choices also play an integral role in beneficial bacteria insufficiency, as these bacteria require the nourishment from whole-food fiber to thrive. A low-fiber diet not only decreases the amount of beneficial microbes in the gut, but also increases the growth of pathogenic bacteria that thrive in a lower acidic environment.[12] The standard American diet filled with processed carbohydrates and toxic seed oils further contributes to intestinal permeability and the reduction of beneficial microbiota.[13]

Low levels of these important bacteria, whether from birth, from an acute incident, or from poor dietary choices, can impair a wide range of functions and pave the way for further digestive dysfunction.

Phase two: Impaired digestive capacity

You are not what you eat; you are what you actually chemically digest and absorb. If you are unable to chemically digest protein, carbohydrates, or fatty acids, you can become deficient in these macronutrients, as well as in the plethora of nutrients they provide.

Hydrochloric acid

Hydrochloric (stomach) acid is one of the most important components of chemical digestion, and most women are deficient in stomach acid – a condition called hypochlorhydria.

Signs of low stomach acid:

- Burping after meals
- Heartburn or a stomach burning sensation
- Reflux or gastroesophageal reflux disease (GERD)

- Bloating shortly after meals
- Loss of taste for animal proteins
- Sense of excess fullness after meals
- Low appetite (especially in the morning)
- Sleepy after meals
- Fingernails that easily break, chip, or peel
- Slow or no hair grow
- Stomach pains and cramps
- Undigested food in the stool

The pharmaceutical industry would have us believe that high stomach acid is the cause of conditions like reflux and heartburn, and that levels rise as we age, since these symptoms tend to increase with age, but a quick look at the scientific literature surrounding this topic reveals that the opposite is true.[14] The use of neutralizing or buffering antacids and acid-suppressing medications can inhibit the absorption of protein, minerals, and a few crucial vitamins, leading to malnutrition.

Bacterial imbalances in the stomach, including for helicobacter pylori (H. pylori), commonly change the pressure of the environment of the stomach. While H. pylori is a normal bacteria found in the stomach lining for most of us, the mechanism by which the bacteria burrows into the lining of the stomach can reduce stomach-acid production, in addition to changing the pressure of the stomach. This change in pressure in combination with the mechanical churning of the stomach in an attempt to facilitate digestion leads to the opening of the sphincter located at the top of the stomach opening, allowing stomach acid to re-enter the esophagus to cause heartburn, indigestion, and even reflux. These are signs typically thought of as "high stomach acid," even though the acid may actually be insufficient. These bacterial overgrowths stem from inadequate stomach acid in the first place.

Fortunately, hydrochloric-acid (HCI) replacement supplementation, such as betaine hydrochloride, is safe and affordable and can be used to enhance digestion and improve overall digestive capacity. Here's how you can use an HCl supplement at home to support digestion:

- Utilizing as low of a betaine chloride dosage as possible, you'll work to slowly increase your dosage per meal to find your bioindividual tolerance. The dosage per capsule/tablet we recommend is 150 mg of betaine HCl.
- Take HCl mid-meal, after at least a few bites of your food.
- Begin by taking 1 HCl supplement (150-mg betaine hydrochloride tablet) per meal. As long as you don't feel adverse digestive symptoms, continue taking 1 HCl with every meal for 1 week and then increase the dose to 2 per meal. Adverse digestive symptoms may include: a warm sensation in the stomach, heartburn, gurgling in the stomach, reflux, diarrhea, or any other digestive changes that are outside of what is normal for you.
- Continue taking 2 per meal for 1 week and, as long as no adverse digestive symptoms have arisen, then increase the dose to 3 per meal. Continue this process of increasing the dosage slowly until you achieve tolerance, which is the point at which you experience adverse digestive symptoms.
- If and when any adverse digestive symptoms arise, cut back the dose to the previous dose where there were no adverse symptoms present. For example, if at four 150-mg tablets per meal there are no symptoms, but when the dose is increased to five 150-mg tablets per meal, there are adverse digestive symptoms, then go back to 4 tablets per meal. If no adverse digestive symptoms are present at that point, 4 tablets per meal is the optimal dose.
- Over time, and as the body increases its own capacity to produce HCl, the dose that initially worked well may also begin to trigger symptoms, which is the indication that it is time to reduce the dose again, to 3 tablets per meal in this example.
- It is critical to find your upper threshold (the highest dose you can handle) in order to ensure you are fully digesting and absorbing your food.

Note that you should not introduce supplemental HCI if you regularly experience heartburn or reflux. Instead, you'll want to reduce the incidence of these symptoms by doing the following:

1. Avoid foods that weaken the lower esophageal sphincter, such as chocolate, coffee, mints (peppermint and spearmint), sugar, alcohol, onions, and foods to which you are allergic.
2. Avoid foods that irritate the esophagus, such as citrus fruits and juices, tomato-based foods, spicy foods, coffee, and carbonated beverages.
3. Utilize an upper GI healing agent such as aloe vera juice, slippery elm, or marshmallow root, 20–30 minutes ahead of meals to soothe the mucous membranes of the upper GI tract before a meal is introduced.

If you do not experience heartburn or reflux symptoms for at least 2 weeks, you can try to introduce a low dosage of betaine hydrochloride (150 mg is recommended) at each meal, watching carefully for the presence of any adverse digestive symptoms that may indicate a longer duration of upper GI healing support is needed.

Vagal toning exercises and supporting healthy nervous system function can also be crucial to support reducing heartburn and promoting healthy stomach acid production.

Bile

Bile production and release are facilitated by the liver and gallbladder. Bile is produced in the hepatocytes of the liver before being stored in the gallbladder and then released into the duodenum of the small intestine to emulsify fats and escort neutralized toxins out of the body. This release of bile from the gallbladder is only stimulated when fatty acids are present in the diet and enter the small intestine. Bile also plays a key role in stimulating peristalsis (which moves food through your digestive system), so constipation is often a result of biliary dysfunction.

Dysfunction in the biliary tree can result from a number of factors, including biliary dyskinesia (or a disturbance in the coordination of contraction of the biliary ducts and/or a reduction in the speed of the emptying into the small intestine), stagnant bile due to poor quality dietary fats, bile insufficiency due to inadequate quantities of dietary fats, and cholestasis.

Gallbladder stones can also contribute to biliary issues and are typically formed from cholesterol, pigments, and other constituents in bile to form hard particles. It's important to understand here that while dysfunction in the gallbladder can impact digestion, dysfunction in the gallbladder often comes as a result of dysfunction further north, in the liver.

Without adequate fat digestion, deficiency in fat-soluble vitamins such as A, D, K, and E is inevitable, as these vitamins are carried by fatty acids throughout the body. Fatty acids, especially cholesterol, are also crucial in the development and production of sex hormones.

Without fat digestion, endocrine imbalances can manifest as menstrual irregularities, weight problems, dry skin, fatigue, increased sensitivity to cold or heat, estrogen dominance, and PCOS, just to name a few.

Signs of poor bile production:

- Stomach upset by fatty or greasy goods
- Greasy or shiny stools
- Stools that float
- Nausea (especially after eating fatty foods)
- Light or clay-colored stools
- Gallbladder attacks
- Hemorrhoids
- Constipation
- Feeling of incomplete bowel emptying
- Abdominal tightness

- Heartburn
- Bloating
- Constipation
- Pain under the rib cage, on the right side
- Jaundice – yellowing of the eyes and skin
- Gallstones

Here are some ways to support biliary function and bile production:

- Consume healthy fats with each meal, such as coconut, avocado, butter, ghee, nuts, and seeds
- Avoid or reduce the consumption of vegetable oil, canola oil, and seed oils
- Regularly consume beets or beet kvass, which can be helpful in stimulating bile flow and thinning the bile.
- Introduce dandelion greens to your diet, as these support bile production and encourage fat metabolism
- Consume plenty of dark leafy greens and cruciferous vegetables, which support natural detoxification of the liver

Pancreatic enzymes

The pancreas is both an endocrine and exocrine gland, in that it produces hormones to assist in the regulation of blood sugar, while also producing digestive juices to assist in the chemical breakdown of food. The enzymes contained in pancreatic juices assist in the digestion of a wide range of nutrients, including proteins, fatty acids, and carbohydrates.

Signs of insufficient pancreatic enzymes:

- Food in stool
- Gas
- Bloating

Other considerations for improving digestive capacity:

- Sit down when eating.
- Eat meals undistracted by phones, TV, computers, or other screens.
- Take 3–5 deep, belly breaths before taking your first bite of food.
- Chew food slowly and thoroughly to support saliva production and mechanical digestion.
- Take a 10–15 minute walk following a meal.

Phase three: Pathogen overgrowth

Chronic pathogenic infections, such as yeast, viruses, bacteria, and parasites, can all be driving factors for chronic immune challenges, which ultimately lead to immune dysfunction. In some cases, this looks like a compromised immune system, while in others, it can look like autoimmunity. It's important to understand that the body makes no mistakes, and while conditions like autoimmunity are often framed as the body being confused and the immune system attacking its own cells, I want to encourage you to think of these types of immune dysfunction differently. What if instead of being confused, the immune system knows exactly what it's doing and is attacking cells in the organs where dysfunction and toxicity exist in an innately intelligent attempt to restore balance?

These pathogens overgrow as a result of toxin exposure and create immune dysfunction and fight back against your immune system while depleting important nutrients. Remember that most of the immune system resides in the GI tract, and when there is an infection, the immune system works hard to fight against it. Initially it may be over-stimulated to fight back, while over time you may notice that your immune system is unable to fight back against infections. The immune function is then compromised and unable to keep up with demands as these pathogens activate the immune system long term.

An overgrowth of pathogens (whether bacterial, fungal, or parasitic) also promotes the production of biofilm. Biofilm is a protective mechanism that organisms in our GI tract use to evade the immune system and prolong their lives. Biofilms are a normal part of everyday life. When you wake up in the morning and have a film across your teeth, that's a biofilm. In the GI tract, these are particularly important, as they promote the overgrowth of pathogens and can encapsulate toxins.

Microorganisms in the GI tract produce a gooey substance to create a network of sugars, proteins, and nucleic acids (such as DNA). You can think of this as like a protective goo that can sequester nutrients such as minerals, but also harmful substances like heavy metals. Over time, more layers of biofilm build up, creating a bulbous, three-dimensional "community" or complex of microorganisms embedded and protected in this biofilm matrix. Multiple species can inhabit the same biofilm matrix, sharing nutrients and genetic material, and changing the environment around them to be more resistant to both immune cells and antimicrobials.[15]

Pathogens can also create dysregulation with the immune system, creating more immune responses to food and even autoimmune reactions. This can result in changes in immune function, either making the system depressed and unable to keep up with demands or causing systematic upregulation, thereby creating new reactions to various foods and exposures. This is where autoimmune conditions come into play.

Our microbiomes are shared, meaning that the microbiome of our gut is also shared with our reproductive tract. Due to the close proximity, it's not uncommon for pathogens to migrate from the anus to the vaginal tract, resulting in yeast infections, UTI's, and even parasitic infections of the uterus.

Elevated levels of bacteria can contribute to elevations in beta-glucuronidase, a liver enzyme involved in one of the most important Phase II conjugation liver pathways for the excretion of carcinogens, lipid-soluble hormones, and steroid hormones. Its purpose is to create a bond between toxins and hormones targeted for excretion. When bacteria is elevated, these bonds become broken and these toxins (both exogenous and endogenous) can be recirculated, creating more toxicity in the body.

All of these factors can lead to intestinal permeability, more commonly known as "leaky gut." Under normal circumstances, these membranes are extremely selective about what enters the bloodstream. When operating normally, food particles are chemically digested and pathogens/toxins are prevented from directly entering the bloodstream. When gut infections occur, the tissues are inflamed and leaky gut or permeability occurs. The villi in the intestinal tract become more like highways rather than selectively permeable membranes, thus allowing undigested food particles, pathogens, and toxins to enter the bloodstream unhindered. This can result in more frequent sickness, increased toxin absorption, and experiencing more food sensitivities over time. While it's easy to blame food when this happens, food is not the problem. When we resolve the pathogenic load, we resolve the leaky gut, and food sensitivities rebalance as the immune system balance is restored.

There are three primary types of pathogens to consider when it comes to imbalances in the microbiome.

Bacteria

In addition to beneficial bacteria, there are also pathogenic and inflammatory bacteria that normally reside in the GI tract at low levels. Many of these bacteria are not problematic when present in small amounts and are considered a normal part of a diverse microbiome, but they can create severe inflammation and release endogenous toxins when they overgrow.

For instance, the Streptococcus species is a normal bacteria found in the GI tract. At low levels, it's expected to be found in microbiome analysis, but at elevated levels it can cause loose stools and intestinal inflammation.

Other pathogenic bacteria can create a wide range of symptom presentations depending on the strains that are elevated as well as the combination of pathogens present.

Symptoms associated with bacterial overgrowth include:

- Abdominal pain and cramps
- Bloating and abdominal distention
- Nausea
- Diarrhea
- Constipation
- Gas
- Fatigue
- Intolerance to sulfurous foods (garlic, onions)
- Foul (rotten egg) smelling gas
- Histamine intolerance

Yeast

Generally, yeast is a harmless commensal, meaning it exists at a normal level in all human intestinal tracts. The presence of yeast under normal circumstances regulates the intestines and protects them from pathogens and other things that can damage the intestinal lining. They also modulate different parts of the immune system.

However, yeast can become pathogenic because of factors that include poor diet,[16] inadequate digestive secretions,[17] a weakened immune system,[18] corticosteroid use, oral contraceptives or estrogen replacement,[19] or antibiotic use.[20] As a result, yeast can spread beyond the GI tract into the nose and sinuses, mouth, vagina, and bladder.

Antibiotic overuse is one of the leading factors for the overgrowth of yeast in the microbiome, as it's been well-documented that the destruction of both beneficial and harmful bacteria occur during antibiotic use. This destruction of beneficial bacteria leads the way for normal yeast in the microbiome to overgrow as the opportunity arises.

Hormonal birth control is another key factor in the overgrowth of yeast for women. Research shows that elevated estrogen levels can increase yeast overgrowth risk due to the mechanism in which estrogen raises blood sugar levels that can feed yeast in the GI tract.[21] Most hormonal birth control options utilize exogenous estrogen to facilitate the disruption of a woman's ovulation, and even progesterone-only contraceptives can burden the liver and its ability to metabolize estrogens effectively - leading to estrogen excess even without the introduction of exogenous estrogens.

Experts believe that the susceptibility to yeast overgrowths while using hormonal contraceptives is due to the negative impact on gut microbiota diversity, which can provide an environment for species like Candida to thrive. The estrogen component of these contraceptives promotes fungal virulence by enabling Candida albicans, in particular, to avoid the actions of the innate immune system.[22]

Candida is one of the most recognized yeasts that overgrow in the GI tract. The genus Candida is made up of over 200 species of fungi, but Candida albicans is the most common fungal pathogen in the GI tract that can result in vaginal yeast infections, diarrhea, brain fog, fatigue, and muscle or joint pain.

Candida overgrowths can be protective in response to toxin exposure. In the case of both heavy metals and radioactive chemicals, Candida can begin to proliferate as a protective mechanism to prevent the recirculation of these toxins systemically. This is especially true for cases of recurrent Candida overgrowth

Symptoms associated with yeast and fungal overgrowth include:

- Sugar cravings
- Alcohol cravings
- History of athlete's foot or nail fungus
- Fatigue

- Feeling of being "drained"
- Acne, especially on back and shoulders
- Feeling drunk without consuming alcohol
- Poor memory
- Depression
- Numbness, burning or tingling in appendages
- Muscle aches
- Pain and/or swelling in joints
- Abdominal pain
- Constipation
- Diarrhea
- Bloating
- Troublesome vaginal discharge or yeast infections
- Headaches
- Inability to concentrate
- Itchy skin and/or rashes
- Sinus issues
- Oral thrush (white-coated tongue)
- Urinary tract infections (and vaginal yeast infections)

Dietary factors, such as a diet with excess carbohydrate consumption or blood sugar dysregulation, are key factors for feeding these fungal pathogens and must be considered as part of a rebalancing protocol. An anti-fungal diet can be helpful for reducing nourishment of yeast, which is primarily sugar.

Many anti-fungal diets are extremely restrictive to carbohydrates and sugars. While this is certainly effective, it can be challenging when the goal is conception, as carbohydrates are required for the healthy production of hormones. Low carbohydrate intake has been linked to hypothyroidism,[23] increased cortisol output, and impaired overall endocrine function at the level of the brain.[24] This means that balancing blood sugar is crucial, which we'll discuss in more depth in Chapter 16, but consuming adequate fiber-rich carbohydrates is an important part of your diet with the goal of healthy hormonal function, regardless of yeast overgrowth concerns.

Use this anti-fungal diet as a guide for reducing the foods that feed yeast, while promoting the foods that stabilize blood sugar and nourish beneficial gut microbiota.

Reduce or remove the following foods:

- Refined and simple sugars, including barley malt, artificial sweeteners, maple syrup, and chocolate.
- Processed/refined flours and simple carbohydrates
- Excess fruit intake (focus on low-sugar fruits like berries, green apple, lemon, and lime)
- Alcohol
- Kombucha
- Foods high in yeast, mold, or fungus, such as cheese, dried fruits, melons, peanuts, corn, rye, and coffee not tested for mycotoxins
- Hot dogs, salami, all processed lunch meats
- Baked goods, including bread
- Condiments such as BBQ sauce and ketchups that contain added sugar

Include these foods daily:

- Animal proteins (grass-fed, pasture-raised chicken and turkey, lamb, beef, fish, pork, eggs)
- Nuts and seeds (soaked and dehydrated are best)
- Low glycemic vegetables and leafy greens, especially cruciferous vegetables
- Cultured vegetable foods
- Raw, unpasteurized apple cider vinegar
- Fresh, organic herbs
- Ghee, butter, or coconut oil
- Unprocessed oils (olive, avocado, sesame)
- Stevia, monk fruit, erythritol, or xylitol (if tolerated)
- Be mindful of carbohydrate intake (more help in Chapter 16)

In addition to promoting a balanced diet mindful of carbohydrate and sugar intake, promoting beneficial bacteria, and removing contributing factors for the overgrowth of yeast, antifungal agents can be supportive in rebalancing these organisms in the GI tract.

Antifungal agents include:

- Goldenseal
- Black walnut
- Echinacea
- Grapefruit seed extract
- Allicin (active ingredient in garlic)
- Caprylic acid
- Turmeric
- Olive leaf
- Tea tree
- Cloves
- Oregano leaf
- Calendula
- Neem
- Forsythia
- Pau d'arco

Parasites

Though parasites are often thought of as a third-world country problem, we all have parasites of different kinds residing in our digestive tracts. They are a normal and sometimes protective part of our gut microbiome and include protozoa and helminths.

There are between 75,000 and 300,000 estimated helminth species and an inestimable number of protozoa. Humans are hosts to at least 370 helminths and protozoa, and we have evolved alongside these organisms, which date back to 9,000 years ago, as hookworms have been found in archaeological sites in North and South America.[25]

Today, however, parasites are considered one of the major contributors to the global disease load. For example, in 2013, there were over 1-million deaths due to parasite infections.[26]

Historically, many cultures have routinely conducted parasite eradication, knowing that these organisms can cause significant health issues when able to overpopulate our bodies.

There are several factors that increase susceptibility to parasitic overgrowths, including age (as children are more susceptible), immune system function based on co-infections, immunosuppressant medications, or a compromised immune system, dietary and lifestyle choices that increase exposure to parasites, low hydrochloric acid and enzyme production, and gut dysbiosis that creates a toxic environment in which parasites thrive.

Parasite infections may be one of the most overlooked infections of our generation, with direct connections to reproductive health. There are reports that some protozoa, helminths, and fungi may impair women's reproductive capacity, causing deformities of the genital tract so that conception is impossible, or, if conception does occur, normal implantation and development of placenta are impossible.[27] In conditions like endometriosis, parasites can invade the uterus and endometrial lining, and migrate into the reproductive system to contribute to infertility.[28] Parasites have been observed in cervicovaginal smears and can infect these areas and form cysts, which can play a part in the disease being mistaken as endometriosis.[29]

Parasitic infections also contribute to infertility through their role in iron anemia. All forms of life require iron to grow and survive, and this includes parasites. Research indicates that when hookworms are deprived of iron, they are not able to grow into their full adult form.[30] Many intracellular parasites lack iron-storage protein and therefore, require a constant source of iron to stay alive.[31] Once infected, humans become this reliable and consistent source, which results in iron-deficient anemia.

These organisms can also cause conditions in other organs, such as the biliary tract,[32] pancreas,[33] skin,[34] brain,[35] and immune system.[36]

Symptoms associated with parasitic overgrowth include:

- Digestive issues (constipation, diarrhea, alternation of both)
- Gas
- Bloating
- Mucus in stool
- Chronic fatigue syndrome (CFS)
- Intestinal permeability
- Allergies
- Chronic ear and sinus infections
- Rashes
- Insomnia or waking up multiple times during the night
- Teeth grinding at night, jaw pain or clenching
- Joint pain
- Anemia
- PMS
- Chronic Candida
- Endocrine disruption
- Restless sleep
- Poor nutrient absorption
- Muscle and joint pain
- Muscle twitches
- Eye floaters
- Headaches, migraines
- Seizures
- Constant hunger
- Foul smelling stools
- Anal itching, especially at night
- Mood issues (anxiety, depression, hyperactivity)
- Skin issues (acne, eczema, psoriasis, hives, etc.)
- Wheezing and coughing
- Unexplained dizziness, weakness
- Brain fog

Common types of parasitic infections

Below are some of the most common types of parasitic infections seen in my practice. While some of them are visible to the naked eye and can be seen during the process of eradication, many are not. The big parasites can be just as harmful to your health as the small ones. There are three primary types of parasites: protozoa, helminths, and ectoparasites.

Most parasites are single-celled protozoa, and they can invade any single cell in our bodies. Protozoa reproduce and multiply by duplicating themselves like a bacteria or virus. Most protozoa are too small to be seen with the naked eye.

Helminths, also commonly known as worms, live in the gastrointestinal tract, blood, lymphatic system, and other tissues. They are multicelled organisms that can live on or inside the body.

Ectoparasites can be transmitted from ticks, fleas, lice, mites, bed bugs, or any other biting insect (including mosquitos). They live on the surface of the human skin or feed off the skin.

Ascaris (roundworms)

Ascaris (also known as roundworms) are one of the most common helminths and are typically found within the small intestine. Ascaris can harbor bacteria such as Lyme, Lyme co-infections, heavy metals, Candida, mold and viruses. The eggs of ascaris are found in feces and soil. Ascaris can also be transmitted via animals, such as through contaminated pork. Ascaris affect vitamin C in the organs where they infect.

Ascaris are thin, like pencils. They can multiply rapidly; a female worm can produce up to 200,000 eggs a day. Roundworms can be up to 3 feet long.

Ascaris and other roundworms can cause physical blocking of the GI tract, leading to bloating, bowel obstructions, and more. They have also been known to block the pancreatic duct and be a cause of pancreatitis. This is largely due to their size.

Common symptoms of the presence of ascaris include:

- Abdominal pain and inflammation
- General weakness
- Teeth grinding
- Drooling while sleeping
- Body itching
- Liquid bowel movements (sometimes with visible worms) and/or constipation
- Fatigue
- Mitochondrial dysfunction
- Eczema
- Acne (especially around the jaw/neck)
- Seizures
- Depression
- Schizophrenia
- Night sweats

Pinworms (roundworms)
Another commonly recognized type of helminth is the pinworm. Adult pinworms are generally 1/4 to 1/2 inch in length. The most common symptom of infection is anal itching, particularly at night, as worms migrate to the host's anal area to lay their eggs. They can also cause vaginal itching, insomnia, irritability, teeth grinding, restlessness, and occasional stomach pain or nausea.

Pinworms are common among school-age children, as they are easily spread from child to child. In these cases, they're treated with an oral antiparasitic medication, but it's recommended that the entire family undergo treatment, due to the contagious nature of these pathogens.

The acceptance of pinworms as a normal occurrence in childhood is just one way we can see parasites in our society as a normal concern, but we often miss these same concerns for women during the conception phase when they are struggling to conceive.

Strongyloides (threadworms)
Strongyloides are often referred to as "threadworms" and can invade any part of the body. Most commonly, they infect the small intestines. They can also cause masses in the breasts, tumors, and cysts within the brain and can invade the sinus cavity.

Common symptoms includes:

- Abdominal pain, diarrhea or constipation
- Food allergies especially dairy
- Migraines and headaches
- Depression and anxiety
- Pulmonary symptoms
- Eosinophilia (elevated eosinophils, a type of white blood cell)
- Fatigue
- Disruption of bowel mucosa
- Rashes

Toxoplasma
Toxoplasma is a protozoan parasite that can be transmitted via contaminated food, water, soil, from mother to child, or through sexual contact. It is also commonly found in cats and cat feces, (which is why when you are pregnant, it's a common recommendation that you should not clean a cat's litter box). Toxoplasma can cause serious complications for pregnant women and in people with weakened immune systems. This is another example of the acknowledgement of the presence of parasites in our culture and their potential dangers.

Toxoplasma can live in the body inactively and become reactivated if the person becomes immunosuppressed. Toxoplasma is linked to behavioral issues like anger, OCD, autism, schizophrenia, brain lesions, and more.[37] It's also known to cause risky behavior, and many ER physicians and nurses see an increase in motorcycle accidents around the time of a full moon, when parasites are at their most active, resulting in increased symptomology in their hosts. Furthermore, all donated organs, such as the liver, are tested for Toxoplasma gondii in the deceased,[38] as it's considered a commonplace concern. It's estimated that around 25% of Americans are infected with toxoplasmosis.[39]

Common symptoms may include:

- Muscle aches and pain
- Fever
- Headaches
- Swollen lymph nodes
- Malaise
- Inflammation of the lung
- Heart palpitations
- Fatigue
- Cognitive stress and seizures
- Depression
- Anxiety
- Inflammation of the eyes and other vision issues
- Chronic pink eye
- Loss of coordination
- Encephalitis
- Shortness of breath
- Weight loss
- Loss of appetite and/or diarrhea

Giardia (protozoa)

Giardia is a parasite that colonizes the small intestine. It is transmitted through contaminated water. Giardia has been found in many forms of water, including unfiltered tap water, lakes, streams, and recreational water. It is protected by an outer shell that allows it to survive outside the body for long periods of time. Giardia is also resistant to chlorine and is often transmitted through water sources, even when those sources contain chlorine for antimicrobial effects.[40]

Common symptoms include:

- Diarrhea
- Vomiting
- Flatulence
- Abdominal distension
- Impediments to nutrient absorption
- Fatigue
- Gas
- Nausea
- Stomach cramps
- Dehydration
- Failure to thrive (children)
- Lactose intolerance and dairy sensitivities

Taenia (tapeworms)

Tapeworms are what most people think of when they think of parasites living in our intestinal tracts. These worms are notorious for stealing our nutrients and cause drastic health changes, but are typically considered rare in the United States despite their presence worldwide. Tapeworms can cause long-term nutrient deficiencies, especially for vitamin B12.

Common symptoms include:

- Insatiable hunger
- Weight loss
- Nausea
- Fatigue
- Stomach cramps
- Diarrhea

Symptoms are often mild and go on for long periods of time being mistaken for common digestive problems. Cystic larval infections often cause no symptoms. They may be visible as lumps under your skin, or they may make themselves known by causing complications to your internal organs. In more severe cases, the larvae can cause itching skin, hives, coughing, chest pain, headaches, seizures, confusion, and blockages to various digestive organs.[41]

Tapeworms can range from 4 inches to over 12 feet in length, have a lifespan of up to 25 years, and can produce up to 300,000 eggs per day.

Protective mechanisms

Now that you're terrified about the critters living in your intestines, it's important to keep in mind that these organisms are a normal part of our microbiome, and we expect them to be present. We all have parasites, and in many cases, they are protective, particularly against toxicity in our lives.

One study showed that those with helminth infections were less likely to experience dyslipidemia, metabolic syndrome, diabetes, and atherosclerotic cardiovascular disease, while those who underwent anti-helminth treatment saw rises in these metabolic disorders.[42] This means that parasites are good for us, and we should leave them alone, right?

The answer isn't quite that simple. Parasites, particularly helminths, respond to environmental stressors and pollutants.[43] In our body, this looks like the toxins we come into on a daily basis and accumulate over the course of our lives. Their presence (and overgrowth) is a response to toxin burden. Parasites are known to harbor heavy metals,[44] mold, Lyme,[45] and other toxins.

Remember that parasites are reliant on us as hosts to survive. When toxin burden increases, their presence increases to prevent the circulation of these damaging toxins. As a result, during anthelmintic treatments, our toxin burden begins to recirculate and without adequate elimination and reduction of exposure to these toxins, it makes sense that metabolic disorders would increase as a result of the protective mechanism being removed.

Does this mean that parasites are the real problem? No, it means that toxin burden is the real problem, and while these organisms may certainly require eradication, we need to also ensure that the reason they are overgrowing in the first place is also under consideration.

It's for this reason that zero parasites is not the goal. If they are overgrowing and cause symptom onset, then removal is a crucial part of healing and reducing stress on the body, but we want to maintain these organisms in our internal terrain to keep us safe in our exceedingly dangerous and toxic world.

Reducing exposure sources

In the name of preventing overgrowth of these organisms, reducing exposure sources is an important part of promoting overall balance in the microbiome. Let's talk about ways you can reduce exposure and support healthy levels of parasites in your gut microbiome.

Ways to reduce exposure to parasites and support healthy levels:

- Limit the consumption or raw or uncooked pork, beef, fish, crabs, and crayfish.
- Avoid drinking unfiltered tap water, as it is not cleared of parasites.[46 47]
- Be mindful of sexual transmission possibilities.[48 49]
- Avoid letting your pets lick you in the mouth and sleep in your bed.[50]
- Prevent bug bites when possible, as ectoparasites are transmitted through all biting insects (ticks, mosquitos, lice, etc.) [51 52]
- Avoid touching contaminated surfaces, such as public toilets.
- Avoid blood transfusions when possible. (The American Red Cross only tests for Babesia and Trypanosoma as parasitic infectious diseases in blood donations.)[53]

- Consider parasite eradication if needed prior to conception, as these organisms can be passed from mother to child in utero,[54 55 56] as well as through breastmilk.[57]
- Consume plenty of anti-parasitic foods (listed in table below).
- Routinely de-worm pets (all).

Anti-Parasitic Foods	
Pineapple	Onion
Papaya seeds	Raw cabbage
Pomegranate	Kelp
Blackberries	Coconut oil
Pomegranate juice	Turmeric
Cranberries	Ginger
Garlic (raw especially)	Clove
Citrus fruit	Psyllium husk
Carrots (raw)	Flax seeds
Sweet potatoes	Pumpkin seeds (raw and sprouted are best)
Winter squash	

Many herbs and spices are anti-parasitic in nature and have been part of traditional diets for centuries to support the routine clearing of parasites from the microbiome.

Anti-parasitic herbs include:

- Anise
- Barberry
- Black walnut
- Clove oil
- Coconut oil
- Curcumin
- Curled mint
- Ginger
- Goldthread
- Goldenseal
- Grapefruit seed extract
- Neem
- Oregano oil
- Oregon grape
- Turmeric
- Wormwood

As you may have noticed, there are several symptoms that overlap between pathogens, which is why comprehensive testing via stool analysis is often helpful for determining a path forward to resolve dysbiosis. The stool tests we most commonly use are the GI-MAP from Diagnostic Solutions and the Gut Zoomer from Vibrant America, although there are many others on the market that can help assess microbiome status.

Remember that many of these pathogens utilize biofilms effectively, to evade detection, so a combination of stool testing and blood chemistry (to look at immune function via a complete blood count with differential) is the best way to comprehensively assess for pathogenic burden in the body, in addition to considering symptom presentation.

A note on pleomorphism

Microbes that normally reside in the gut are known to be pleomorphic, which means that they have the ability to alter their morphology, form, reproductive capacity, and other metabolic behavior in response to environmental inputs and changes. As we discussed in the connection between heavy metals, chemicals, and pesticides and their role in altering the gut microbiome, this means that exposure to toxicity can alter the state of our gut microbiome, allowing for pathogens to overgrow and cause symptoms. From this perspective, while eradication and rebalancing of the gut are crucial to removing the burden on hormonal health and fertility, removing and addressing toxicity is crucial to ensuring that future pathogens are mitigated.

Chapter 14
Hypothyroidism and Revitalizing Function

CORE PRINCIPLE SEVEN: Assess for subclinical hypothyroidism and support function as needed

Hypothyroidism is incredibly common among women, with 15% of women experiencing clinical hypothyroidism.[1 2] Subclinical hypothyroidism levels are those in which hormone levels are considered "normal" but may fall outside of optimal ranges, giving you symptoms of hypothyroidism and negatively impacting the ability to conceive.

Hypothyroidism can cause infertility by preventing ovulation and impairing cellular division in the event that fertilization of an egg does occur. If you are hypothyroid, you have an elevated risk of miscarriage and may experience elevated levels of prolactin, making conception even more difficult.

Hypothyroidism's effects on metabolism can also bring on a condition known as luteal phase defect, creating fertility issues because the uterine lining can't build up sufficiently for the embryo to implant. In both men and women, proper thyroid regulation helps facilitate optimal estrogen and testosterone production, which supports a healthy libido.

On the other side of things, hypersecretion of thyroid hormone affects ovulation in females and can result in impotence in males.

Thinking ahead to birth and breastfeeding, thyroid hormones play an integral role in female mammary function. During lactation, they aid in the regulation of both prolactin and oxytocin.

Whether you think thyroid function is impacting fertility or not, assessing function in these areas will ensure that no stone is left unturned and provide you a baseline ahead of pregnancy, as thyroid shifts are not uncommon postpartum.

What causes hypothyroidism?

Many women share the sentiment that thyroid issues are genetic and run in their family, but the truth is that the presentation of thyroid dysfunction is often the result of other systemic imbalances, dietary choices, emotional stress, and deficiencies that occur generationally.

Estrogen dominance is a leading factor for hypothyroidism. This may be why more females than males are affected with thyroid imbalances, but this is also likely related to estrogen-mimicking environmental toxins and other endocrine disruptors that women are more likely to come in contact with in their daily life. Addressing toxin burden is essential for restoring balance in hypothyroidism.

Heavy metals can also aggravate the thyroid by inhibiting deiodinases, which are the primary enzymes responsible for the conversion of thyroid hormones into and out of their active form to properly regulate levels systemically.[3] Mercury is one of the most potent and dangerous heavy metals that impact thyroid function, contributing to an increased risk of developing an autoimmune disease that impacts the thyroid, known as Hashimoto's thyroiditis.[4 5] Mercury can be stored in the thyroid in place of iodine, rendering the thyroid unable to produce these hormones at adequate levels.[6 7] Mercury has one of the greatest impacts on thyroid function, with off-gassing from dental work containing this heavy metal impacting the thyroid directly due to its close geographic proximity. Mercury can create a confusing symptom picture with Hashimoto's where you may experience some hypothyroid symptoms, but also some hyperthyroid symptoms (such as heart palpitations). Bloodwork may also reflect some hypothyroid and hyperthyroid patterns in the same person as a result of the toxicity this metal causes in the thyroid.

If these types of environmental toxins don't directly impact thyroid function, it may be impacted through the effects they have on gut health. The microbiome of the intestinal tract plays an integral role in the conversion of thyroid hormones. Thyroid hormones also play a role in managing the tight junctions of the intestinal tract, so those with hypothyroidism are more likely to experience impaired mucosal health and leaky gut.[8]

At its foundation, our primary thyroid hormone, T4 (thyroxine), is composed of tyrosine and four molecules of iodine. Halogens found in environmental chemicals that contain fluoride, bromide, and chlorine are molecularly similar to iodine, as they all contain the same number of electrons in their outer shell, and as a result can replace iodine in the attempt to produce thyroid hormones.[9]

Blood sugar dysregulation also plays a role in thyroid function, as insulin is required to stimulate deiodinase activity for hormone conversion.[10] Ketogenic diets and carbohydrate deprivation have been shown to inhibit deiodination,[11] with low T3 (triiodothyronine) as a result, which is why these diets aren't recommended for women, especially with conception in mind.

With a full toxic bucket and poor blood sugar regulation comes the susceptibility for illness. These types of infections, whether bacterial, fungal, viral, or parasitic, can invade the thyroid. If the thyroid gland has normal levels of iodine, it's able to utilize iodine's antiseptic properties to kill these pathogens. However, in our society, iodine deficiency is incredibly common. Iodine is one of four minerals we'll discuss required for thyroid function, and these systemic infections further contribute to depletion and thyroid imbalances.

Symptoms associated with hypothyroidism:

- Constipation
- Slower than normal GI motility

- Cold hands and feet
- Fatigue
- Brain fog
- Puffy face
- Swelling and edema
- Muscle cramping
- Muscles tender to the touch
- Increased levels of LDL cholesterol, total cholesterol and triglycerides
- Low heart rate or pulse
- Mental sluggishness
- Depression
- Paresthesia (the sensation known as "pins and needles")
- Cognitive challenges.
- Slow metabolism
- Difficulty losing weight
- Dry skin
- Hair loss

Testing your thyroid

If you're concerned about your thyroid, testing your levels via bloodwork is a good first step for assessment and determining support needs. In fact, this is something I recommend for anyone looking to conceive because of what a crucial role the thyroid plays throughout the conception process and pregnancy.

Assessing thyroid function before conception is also a great preventative measure, as postpartum thyroiditis is a common occurrence following the birth of a child. This is a condition where thyroid function changes as a result of the shift of hormones during the immediate postpartum period. Remember that hormones do not function in a bubble, so when one hormone drops significantly, all of our hormones will be impacted. This is especially true following birth, when the levels of both estrogen and progesterone dip to the lowest levels they will in a woman's life, even including during menopause.

If you have a preconception assessment of thyroid function, you'll have a baseline to compare changes to, in the event things don't feel quite right postpartum, and will be able to monitor them through pregnancy, as they are expected to increase to support fetal development.

Markers to test

If you've ever suspected thyroid imbalances, you may have asked your provider to order labs only to find that "everything came back normal." This is in part due to the fact that conventional medicine only looks at one (sometimes two) markers to assess thyroid function.

The primary marker used to indicate thyroid dysfunction from a conventional perspective is TSH (thyroid stimulating hormone). This is the hormone released by the pituitary gland in the brain to communicate with the thyroid gland to impact the amount of thyroid hormone being produced. This system works on a negative feedback loop, where the pituitary produces more TSH when thyroid hormone levels are low, and less TSH when thyroid hormones are high - or at least that's how it should work.

This means that when you assess TSH, it's possible for this marker to come back within normal range without properly assessing the actual thyroid hormone levels.

This method also assumes that communication between the hypothalamus and pituitary glands is always directly correlated to endocrine output, in this case in the thyroid gland. What I commonly see is that function of the brain has been impacted in women for a number of reasons, including long-term hormonal birth control use, stress, and poor work/life balance, leaving their brain unable to properly communicate with the thyroid. As a result, TSH may be optimal, while their thyroid hormones themselves are low. They simply aren't receiving the communication from the brain to increase levels.

To get a more accurate and comprehensive look at thyroid function, it's always important to also test the thyroid hormones themselves: T4 (thyroxine) and T3 (triiodothyronine) in both their total and free forms. Total forms indicate both the unbound and bound hormone levels. When hormones are bound, they are attached to proteins and unable to impact tissues. Unbound, or free, hormone levels are those that are able to impact tissues.

T4 is the inactive form of thyroid hormone and is the most abundant thyroid hormone. T4 must be converted into T3 to fuel the body's metabolism.

T3 is the active form of thyroid hormone and is approximately four times as potent as T4. T3 is considered the truly active hormone and is necessary to perform the critical functions governed by the thyroid.

When looking at your thyroid levels, you might see that T4 is adequate or even slightly elevated, while T3 is low. This is a conversion issue, as the body is producing adequate hormones levels but struggling to convert them into their active form for use.

The liver is the primary site of thyroid conversion, with 40% of overall conversion occurring there. The liver is responsible for removing toxins and excess hormones from the body, and if the liver has a reduced capacity to detoxify, toxins and excess hormones can negatively impact thyroid hormone conversion. Assessing and supporting liver function in our toxic worlds is of utmost importance for supporting thyroid function.

In addition to their many other roles, gut bacteria also assist in the conversion of inactive T4 into the active form of thyroid hormone, T3. Around 20% of T4 is converted to T3 in the GI tract by healthy gut bacteria, and intestinal dysbiosis can therefore reduce the conversion of T3.

Getting an accurate look at these levels can be helpful for determine if hypothyroidism or hyperthyroidism are contributing to your overall hormonal concerns for fertility.

Functional thyroid ranges

Marker	Functional Range	Indications: Elevated Levels may Indicate	Indications: Suboptimal Levels may indicate
TSH	1.00 - 2.00 mlU/L	• Hypothyroidism • Hashimoto's • Anterior Pituitary Dysfunction • Liver dysfunction • GI dysfunction	• Hyperthyroidism • Heavy Metal Burden • High-dose Thyroid Medication • Hashimoto's • Brain-based Hypothyroidism • Cellular Hypothyroidism
Total T4	7.50 - 8.10 ng/dL	• Hyperthyroidism • Thyroid Hormone Medications • Exogenous Estrogen • Euthyroid Sick Syndrome	• Primary of Secondary hypothyroidism • Thyroid Rx containing Triiodothyronine • Iodine deficiency • Exogenous Androgens • Brain-based Hypothyroidism • Cellular Hypothyroidism
Total T3	90.00 - 168.00 ng/dL	• Hyperthyroidism • Iodine Deficiency	• Primary Hypothyroidism • Selenium Deficiency • Brain-based Hypothyroidism • Cellular Hypothyroidism
Free T4	1.00 - 1.50 ng/dL	• Hyperthyroidism • Hereditary Thyroid resistance • Insulin Resistance • PCOS/elevated Testosterone.	• Primary of secondary Hypothyroidism • T3 Replacement • Iodine Deficiency • Pituitary Dysfunction • Estrogen Dominance • Brain-based Hypothyroidism • Cellular Hypothyroidism
Free T3	3.00 - 3.25 pg/mL	• Hyperthyroidism • Iodine Deficiency	• Primary Hypothyroidism • Selenium Deficiency • Low T3 Syndrome • Brain-based Hypothyroidism • Cellular Hypothyroidism
TPO Antibodies	0.00 - 34.00	• Hashimoto's • Grave's Disease	
TGB Antibodies	0.00 - 0.90	• Hashimoto's • Thyroid Cancer	

If your labs look normal, even by functional standards, but you still suspect hypothyroidism, other cellular imbalances like calcium, potassium, copper or manganese can disrupt how cells are actually able utilize the active T3 hormone. In other words, thyroid dysfunction can happen anywhere within the production, utilization, or communication cascade in the body.

Thyroid supports

Addressing any potential toxicity is the best way to support the thyroid, as toxins not only directly impact thyroid function, but also create distress in other systems of the body that directly impact thyroid health, such as the liver and GI tract. Dealing with toxicity is a crucial step for natural thyroid rebalancing, in addition to direct support.

One of the best ways to support thyroid function is through nutritional supports, as thyroid function and hormone production are heavily reliant on a number of minerals and nutrients that we are commonly deficient in. It's not uncommon to see nutritional support for the thyroid be supportive enough to avoid or reduce the need for thyroid hormone medications.

There are four minerals essential for healthy thyroid function: iodine, selenium, magnesium, and zinc. Most of us are chronically depleted of these minerals due to poor soil quality and depletion of the soil in which produce is grown. As a result, our food is not as nutrient-dense as it once was.

Iodine

Iodine is the primary nutrient needed for the production of thyroid hormones, as iodine is combined with tyrosine for both T4 and T3 production. In addition to its role for the thyroid, iodine is detected in every organ in the body, and low iodine is associated with several health conditions, including cancer.[12 13]

Iodine deficiency is incredibly common in the U.S., and intake has declined over the past 50 years with it being removed from our food supply. Iodine has historically been added to wheat, but has since been replaced with bromine, the gas used to fumigate termites in homes.[13] Well-known for its ability to prevent and reverse goiters, iodine is crucial for the body to regulate metabolism and weight. It's also associated with a range of negative maternal and fetal outcomes at deficient levels.[14]

While consumption has decreased, the ingestion of toxic halogens such as bromine, fluoride, chlorine, and perchlorate has dramatically increased in food, water, medicines, and the environment. These toxic halogens compete with iodine and displace it throughout the body, further leading to depletion.

Iodine deficiency is also linked to ovarian cysts, migraines, insulin resistance, COPD, cardiovascular disease, fibromyalgia, breast fibroids, impaired cognition and memory, and increased occurrence of infections.[15]

The RDA (recommended dietary allowance) for iodine is 150 mcg per day, yet we know the body's physiological need is about 13 mg per day. Getting iodine through food sources is the best way to introduce this nutrient slowly, though supplementation is often useful. Food sources of iodine include:

- Seaweed (kombu kelp and wakame)
- Cod fish
- Raw dairy

Supplementing with iodine is another alternative if you suspect iodine deficiency. The best type of iodine for supplementation is a combination of iodine and potassium iodide. It's important to slowly increase the dosage, watching for detoxification reactions. Many reactions to iodine thought to be allergies or iodism are detoxification reactions, especially when trying to increase iodine too quickly. When bromine, chlorine, and fluorine are mobilized too rapidly, the result can be a detoxification reaction with all the accompanying effects (headache, fatigue, digestive distress, and even full-blown flu-like symptoms).

The most common apparent reason for these reactions is lack of appropriate nutrient synergists, such as selenium. The body can't uptake iodine without selenium, and without selenium, there would be no activation of thyroid hormone. As such, considering both of these minerals together is crucial.

Selenium

Selenium is a critical nutrient responsible for transforming T4 into the more active T3 and may help protect against free radical damage and cancer systemically.[16] A deficiency in selenium can contribute to pain in the muscles and joints,[17] unhealthy hair,[18] and white spots on the fingernails,[19] as well as Hashimoto's disease, if deficiency is chronic.[20]

Food sources of selenium include:

- Brazil nuts
- Fish
- Eggs
- Raw dairy products
- Grass-fed meats

Supplementing with selenium is often necessary in combination with iodine, and supplementing them together is a good strategy for comprehensive thyroid support, nutritionally. Front-loading, or starting with selenium supplementation prior to beginning iodine supplementation, can also reduce the incidence of detoxification reactions.

Zinc

Zinc is necessary for many of the body's processes and most people are chronically deficient in this vital mineral. It's needed for the metabolism of food and nutrients and is involved with triggering over 100 different internal enzymes in metabolism. Zinc is also crucial for the health of the human immune system to properly regulate any infections, whether in the digestive system or otherwise. It also aids growth through its role in protein building and synthesis, and is therefore particularly needed to sustain a healthy pregnancy.

Food sources of zinc include:

- Seafood (particularly oysters)
- Beef and lamb
- Pumpkin seeds
- Mushrooms

Getting zinc from food sources is the best way to get more of this nutrient, as supplementing with zinc can offset other key minerals, such as copper. Below is one of my favorite ways to snack on nutrient-dense oysters that contain high levels of bioavailable zinc in combination with other minerals to ensure a healthy balance is maintained.

Oyster recipe

Canned oysters in oil
Sharp cheddar cheese
Gluten free-cracker
Mustard or hot sauce optional

Magnesium

Magnesium is another key nutrient necessary for proper enzymatic output and conversion of active thyroid hormones. While it's always important to seek out magnesium-rich foods, this mineral has been one of the most impacted by the drastic decline in food-based nutrient sources of magnesium that has occurred over the last century. Magnesium content in vegetables has seen declines from 25—80% since pre-1950 figures.[21] For this reason, it's often difficult, if not impossible, to consume sufficient magnesium exclusively from food.

Supplementation of magnesium is recommended for hypothyroidism, and utilizing the right form of magnesium is essential. Magnesium malate and glycinate, which are stimulating and calming, respectively, are the two best forms. We'll discuss magnesium dosage, timing and more in Chapter 15.

Tyrosine

While tyrosine is not a mineral, it's a crucial nutrient for the production of thyroid hormones. Tyrosine is an amino acid that can also increase enzymatic function for thyroid hormone conversion. Tyrosine is found in chicken, turkey, fish, peanuts, almonds, avocados, bananas, dairy products, and many other foods. Ensuring both the consumption of these foods and chemical digestion (as outlined in our Rebalancing the gut chapter) is crucial for ensuring adequate levels of tyrosine for thyroid health.

PMGs for thyroid healing

Protomorphogens (PMGs) are another great strategy, particularly for those with elevated thyroid antibodies, or a Hashimoto's or Grave's diagnosis. Produced by the nucleus of each cell to regulate growth and function, PMGs are the cellular roadmap for health function, and these nucleoproteins are common to all mammals. The use of PMGs with autoimmunity helps to remove interference to cell repair by distracting autoantibodies away from the tissue, according to Dr. Michael Gaeta.[22] This is also known as the "decoy theory," which states that PMGs can be used to distract antibodies and allow for the thyroid to regenerate and heal.

These PMGs are also beneficial in the symptom relief of many thyroid conditions and are safe to use alongside other therapies, such as hormone replacement medication, without stimulating the thyroid gland the way that herbs can.

Remove gluten

If you have a thyroid issue, you should consider fully removing gluten from your diet. This may seem like a bold and broad statement, but it's founded on the fact that gluten creates molecular mimicry in the body in relation to the thyroid.

Molecular mimicry occurs when the cells of some type of antigen (food, in this case) and the cells of self-tissue look similar enough (due to proteins being in the same sequence) to confuse the immune system, resulting in an attack on self, also known as autoimmunity. For the thyroid, this is known as Hashimoto's, and it results in the production of thyroid peroxidase (TPO) antibodies that attack the cells of the thyroid, breaking them down and inhibiting thyroid hormone production.[23]

At a molecular level, thyroid tissue and gluten are almost identical. This means that if you have positive TPO antibodies or a Hashimoto's diagnosis, every time you eat gluten, not only does your immune system mount a response to the gluten, but it also mounts a parallel response to thyroid tissue, exacerbating the autoimmune damage.

Get rid of gluten in all its forms, and be sure to be mindful of cross-contamination of grains, including rice and corn products. While wheat is the commonly recognized source of gluten, it's important to know that you should also stay away from these lesser-known gluten sources: barley, rye, farina, graham flour, and semolina.

Thyroid medications

Thyroid medications can be incredibly supportive for feeling better, normalizing thyroid levels, and seeing progress in fertility. There's no shame in taking a thyroid medication, even if you're someone who doesn't normally like to take pharmaceuticals. They can mean all the difference in conceiving and carrying to full term.

If you think there's a clinical need for thyroid medication, and you've ordered a thyroid panel on your own, it can be helpful to share that information with your physician, who will ultimately refer you to an endocrine specialist to prescribe the medication.

It's important to monitor your thyroid every 3 months for the duration of your time taking thyroid medication, as things can shift, and you may find yourself inadvertently being over-medicated. Your prescribing physician can help you monitor levels and increase or decrease the dosage as needed.

This is especially important as you may have changes in your health that can impact thyroid function. For instance, if you work on gut health, you may improve your ability to produce and convert thyroid hormones over time, resulting in different needs for support. For some health changes it means reducing dosage, while for others it can mean thyroid medication is no longer needed.

Even if you are introducing exogenous T4 hormones, it's still essential to support the conversion of T4 to T3; otherwise, you may still technically fall into the category of hypothyroidism, despite taking the correct dosage of thyroid medication.

The most commonly prescribed T4 medications are:

- Levothyroxine
- Synthroid
- Unithroid
- Levoxyl
- Tirosint
- Euthyrox

Remember that the two primary sites for thyroid hormone conversion are the liver and intestines, so supporting these areas is vital.

In other cases, T3 medications can provide the active form of thyroid hormone for cells to use, allowing the body to utilize the most potent form of thyroid hormones. These medications are more effective for those with conversion issues, who have normal TSH and T4 but are still experiencing hypothyroidism symptoms.

The most commonly prescribed T3 medications are:

- Armour Thyroid
- Nature Thyroid
- NP Thyroid
- WP Thyroid
- Cytomel
- Liothyronine

Thyroid medication & gluten

While many thyroid medications do not contain gluten, it's especially important to ensure that yours does not, as gluten can further exacerbate thyroid dysfunction, especially if your TPO antibodies are elevated or on the cusp of being flagged high. Levothyroxine is one of the most commonly prescribed medications for hypothyroidism and contains gluten. Cytomel also contains gluten.

Thyroid medications contain other fillers worth knowing about, in case you have sensitivities to these types of foods and want to avoid dyes.

Figure 14.1

Fillers in T3

	GLUTEN	LACTOSE	CORN	SUCROSE	DYES
Armour			X		
Nature-Throid		X			
NP Thyroid		X	X		X
WP Thyroid		X			
Cytomel	X		X	X	
Liothyronine			X*		

*Select manufacturers (liothryonine manufactured by Sigma Pharma has corn)

Fillers in T4

	GLUTEN	LACTOSE	CORN	SUCROSE	DYES
Levothyroxine	X*	X	X*	X*	X
Synthroid		X	X		X
Unithroid		X	X		X
Levoxyl					X
Tirosint					
Euthyrox			X		

*Select manufacturers (for levothyroxine generic, Lannett, and Mylan are gluten free)

Chapter 15
Crucial Nutrient Replenishment

CORE PRINCIPLE EIGHT: Consider nutritional deficiencies associated with infertility and replenish as needed

Never in history has there been a more nutrient-deficient society. Between our depleted soil, poor dietary habits, and compromised digestive systems, we're unable to utilize the nutrients from our food even when we are eating all the right things, leaving us in a compromised state.

Toxicity causes deficiencies by inhibiting the normal conversion of nutrients for use systemically. As a result, when a toxicant inhibits a conversion process, further nutrient deficiencies can result. The impacts to gut dysbiosis further exacerbate nutrient deficiencies by lowering enzyme function and impairing chemical digestion for the absorption of nutrients. As a result, multiple nutrient deficiencies are commonly seen in women struggling to conceive. While this is highly bioindividual, and not all deficiencies noted here will apply to you, these are the areas you'll want to explore and consider for support in the form of food-based nutrition or supplementation.

One of the most impactful factors for nutrient deficiencies in women has come with the overuse of hormonal contraceptives. The era of hormonal birth control found many of us starting on the pill as teenagers and using it for a decade or more before we were ready to start families. Except no one told us about the harmful effects of oral contraceptives. Not only do they effectively shut off the communication from the brain to the endocrine system,[1] making it impossible for us to bring our own hormone production back online when the time is right, but they also deplete us of all the essential nutrients needed to get pregnant.[2]

Did you know that your own hormone production is being completely shut off by hormonal birth control? Or that the chronically high levels of exogenous sex hormones create a negative feedback loop that atrophies your pituitary's ability to communicate with all of your endocrine systems - ovaries, adrenals, and thyroid?

Did you think that you would get pregnant as soon as you stopped taking your contraceptives?

If you feel duped, you're not alone.

Millions of women experience what is now being referred to as post-birth control syndrome, which often results in fertility problems. When we remove the exogenous sex hormones being used in hormonal birth control (no matter what type we used), our body is being asked to produce these hormones on its own again. I was on birth control for over 10 years before learning that I wasn't even having a real period (and neither were you). Menstruation while on hormonal contraceptives is a withdrawal bleed as hormones dip while taking your week off or taking sugar pills, but it is not indicative of having a true cycle.

This means that when you come off birth control, your period might completely disappear. On the other hand, it may suddenly shift and happen more frequently than you'd expect (and come with a wide range of unpleasant symptoms).

Hormonal contraceptives deplete the body of essential nutrients, including folate, vitamin B2, vitamin B6, vitamin B12, vitamin C, and vitamin E, as well as the minerals magnesium, selenium, and zinc. A report from the World Health Organization notes that "the influence of oral contraceptives on nutrient requirements is a topic of high clinical concern and should, therefore, receive great attention."[3]

Hello, thyroid problems. Thanks a lot, birth control.

The good news is that you can support these nutrient deficiencies in a number of ways. Here, I've outlined the top nutrient deficiencies that I see in women who have trouble conceiving or experience miscarriages. I would consider focusing on these nutrients and supplementing where indicated for all women with fertility concerns, regardless of whether or not hormonal birth control has been a part of their story.

B vitamins

While most prenatal vitamins contain B vitamins, they may not be in adequate dosages to support deficiencies or may be in non-bioavailable forms. Utilizing an additional B-complex might be supportive of reducing B vitamins deficiencies. Furthermore, if you have a MTHFR genetic mutation, you must utilize a prenatal vitamin or B-complex that contains the methylated forms of these nutrients, in order to absorb and utilize them.

So how do you know if you have a B vitamin deficiency? If you used birth control at any point in time, you'll want to consider a B-complex vitamin for support. If you have low energy levels and fatigue, you're likely low in B vitamins. If your serum homocysteine is above 7 umol/L, you are likely struggling with methylation capacity and need methylated B vitamins. Imbalances in red blood cell health in bloodwork can also indicate B vitamin deficiencies, which are indicated by the MCV, MCH, and MCHC results in bloodwork.

Folate (also known as vitamin B9) is essential for the health of red blood cells and their role of carrying nutrients throughout the body. It's also incredibly important in the conception process and throughout pregnancy, particularly in the prevention of neural tube issues and to support the development of the brain and spinal cord while in utero.

The type of folate included in prenatal vitamins is one of the most contested issues, and the names folate and folic acid are often used interchangeably, despite the fact that they function differently in the body. Folate is a general term used to describe the many different forms of vitamin B9, including folic acid, dihydrofolate (DHF), tetrahydrofolate (THF), 5, 10-methylenetetrahydrofolate (5, 10-MTHF), and 5-methyltetrahydrofolate (5-MTHF).[4] Folic acid is the synthetic form of folate that is commonly used in supplements and in fortified foods. It's had many studies done to show its effectiveness in pregnancy support, but it is still a synthetic form of folate.[5]

Naturally occurring folate is found in a number of foods, including leafy green vegetables, citrus fruits, beef liver, and beans, which is why having a diet with robust levels of folate is important during pregnancy. That being said, if you have the MTHFR gene variation that makes the biochemical process of absorbing folate more challenging (if not impossible), consuming more folate-rich foods may not achieve the desired goal. Instead, using a prenatal vitamin or B-complex that contains methylated folate, ideally in the 5-MTHF form, will ensure that this step of the biochemical process is undergone to support deficiencies.

Folate isn't the only B vitamin important for fertility, however. Vitamin B6 is critical for egg health,[6] progesterone production,[7] and cervical mucus production and quality to promote fertilization of the egg by holding onto sperm.[8] Vitamin B2 is involved in the ATP production, and is therefore important for mitochondrial function to promote the health of eggs and cellular replication throughout pregnancy. Out of the eight B vitamins we need, five of them (B1, B2, B6, B12, folate, and niacin) are involved in ovulation, and deficiencies are linked to a greater likelihood of anovulation (absence of ovulation), and therefore infertility.[9]

It's always important to remember that B vitamins regulate one another, so supplementing with only one B vitamin, (vitamin B12 is the one most commonly seen), you may be inadvertently causing imbalances in B vitamins rather than supporting depletion.[10] Therefore, utilizing a B-complex vitamin where these nutrients are present in specific ratios is not only easier for you, but also provides more comprehensive support.

Magnesium

As we mentioned in Chapter 14, magnesium is an essential mineral for function of many endocrine glands, but its importance goes far beyond this. Magnesium has many important functions in the body and is needed for more than 300 biochemical reactions. It maintains normal nerve and muscle function, supports the immune system, maintains a regular heartbeat, and provides bone strength. It also helps regulate blood glucose levels and aids in the production of energy, protein synthesis, and nucleic acid synthesis, and is used in the blood clotting mechanism.

Magnesium is essential for the detoxification of environmental chemicals and binds to heavy metals to support elimination.

Symptoms associated with magnesium deficiency:

- Low appetite
- Muscle spasms, twitches, or cramps
- Apathetic mood or depression
- Constipation
- Headaches and migraines
- Excess body odor
- Impaired immune function (frequently sick)
- Chemical sensitivity
- Fatigue and weakness
- Abnormal heart rhythms
- Osteoporosis
- High blood pressure
- Asthma

Fluoride in tap water plays a critical role in depleting magnesium and is a further reason to avoid tap water as your primary source of water. Fluoride seeks out magnesium and binds to it, making magnesium unable to do its job in the body. The magnesium fluoride mineral byproduct is called sellaite. It's nearly insoluble and takes the place of magnesium in hard tissues throughout the body, like bones and cartilage.

Stress and magnesium status are intimately connected. Low magnesium levels have been associated with several stressful conditions, such as photosensitive headache, fibromyalgia, chronic fatigue syndrome, audiogenic stress, cold stress, and physical stress, amongst others.[11] At the same time, stress can lead to increased elimination of magnesium. One study showed that university students had high levels of magnesium excreted through their urine during exam season.[12]

If you're stressed, you burn through and eliminate magnesium at higher rates, and at the same time, magnesium deficiency can contribute to more stress and mental health issues.[13] It's a vicious cycle.

Keep in mind that while we're referring to stress as emotional life stressors, stress includes any types of stressor on the body, including internal infections, blood sugar dysregulation, exercise, and toxin burden. For this reason, it's safe to say we could all use more magnesium in our lives to help combat deficiencies and support healthy stress responses. We may even need more than usual in times of particular stress (high level of training, big work projects, stressful life seasons).

Alcohol consumption further depletes magnesium.[14] Ethanol, the main ingredient in alcohol, works as a magnesium diuretic, pulling magnesium and other electrolytes out of the body through the kidneys. Over time, magnesium levels can be chronically depleted by alcohol alone, and magnesium is often used to treat the mental health impacts of alcoholism.

Adequate stomach acid is essential for the absorption of magnesium in all forms including supplementation, so ensuring optimal stomach acid support is of utmost importance (not only for magnesium, but for all minerals).

Types of magnesium

There are seven different forms of magnesium, and each one of them plays a different role in the body. While some are more stimulating, others are calming. Choosing the type(s) of magnesium that best suit your needs is important for getting the most out of your supplementation.

Magnesium citrate is one of the most common forms of magnesium in supplemental form, but it's often not the best choice for magnesium supplementation. While some studies show that this is the most bioavailable form of magnesium for absorption purposes, it also has a laxative effect that can prevent you from reaching an adequate dose to be effective, while avoiding further depletion via diarrhea.

Form of magnesium	**Best used for**
Magnesium citrate	Laxative effect by retaining water in the colon, can cause dehydration in excess
Magnesium glycinate	Calming effect, supports sleep, well-absorbed and easy on stomach
Magnesium oxide	Laxative effect without dehydration, good for constipation relief and motility
Magnesium malate	Energizing properties, best used in morning, fibromyalgia and chronic fatigue syndrome
Magnesium chloride	Typically used topically to relieve muscle cramps and aches, promotes digestion
Magnesium sulfate	Best used in bath for muscle cramps and aches, found in Epsom salt
Magnesium threonate	Supports brain function, cognition and mood, crosses blood-brain-barrier

My most recommended combination of magnesium forms is magnesium malate in a higher dose in the morning, paired with magnesium glycinate in evening. This provides the best of both worlds to harness the energizing benefits in the morning and still reap the rewards of magnesium's calming effects in the evening to promote deep sleep.

Because we can struggle to get adequate magnesium through dietary sources, I recommend trying a higher therapeutic dose of magnesium. Consuming 6–7 mg per pound of body weight is the ultimate goal.

Omega-3 fatty acids

Omega-3 fatty acids are unsaturated fatty acids that include eicosapentaenoic acid (EPA) and docosahexaenoic acid (DHA). These fats are important for the membrane of every cell in the body and are anti-inflammatory to support appropriate inflammation levels.

While also important for fatty acid consumption, omega-6 fatty acids are often imbalanced with these essential acids. Think of omega-6 fatty acids as pro-inflammatory and omega-3 fatty acids as anti-inflammatory. Having the ability to inflame when needed it important – in fact, ovulation is an inflammatory event – but when the body is chronically inflamed without the ability to pump the breaks on inflammation due to lack of omega-3 fatty acids, inflammation can put stress on the body that contributes to hormonal imbalances and typically suboptimal sex hormone levels. The ideal ratio of omega-6s to omega-3s is 4:1, which equates to consuming 1 gram of omega-3s for every 4 grams of omega-6s.[15] Getting this ratio of omegas is a challenge given than pro-inflammatory fats are used in nearly all processed foods, resulting in omega consumption around 30:1 omega-6s to omega-3s.

Omega-3s are also important for endocrine function and hormone function by serving as one of the primary building blocks of hormones. Supplementation of omega-3s has been shown to rebalance FSH levels in PCOS cases,[16] as well as reduce the presence of PMS symptoms, including bloating, cramping, and irritability, which speaks to the capacity of omega-3s to support the balance between progesterone and estrogen during a women's cycle.[17] While utilizing omega-3 fatty acids alone is not enough to resolve true insulin resistance, supplementation with these fatty acids has been shown to improve blood sugar regulation, which impacts all hypothalamic-pituitary function and therefore, supports the function of all endocrine glands in the body.[18]

Sources of omega-6 fatty acids:

- Canola oil
- Vegetable oil
- Sunflower oil
- Safflower oil
- Soy & soybean oil
- Sesame oil
- Corn oils
- Nuts
- Seeds
- Grapeseed oil
- Cottonseed oil
- Margarine (from vegetable oils)
- Conventionally raised meats (contain higher levels of omega-6s)

Sources of omega-3 fatty acids:

- Cod liver oil
- Wild caught salmon
- Sardines
- Oysters
- Mackerel
- Herring

By reducing your consumption of omega-6 fatty acids, particularly in processed foods, and increasing the consumption of omega-3 fatty-acid rich foods, you can better support the optimal ratio between these fats. Supplementation is another easy way to consume adequate omega-3 fatty acids. However, most omega-3 fatty acids supplements on the market contain a marginal amount of EPA and DHA, meaning that they are not as beneficial as they may seem. In order to get adequate levels of omega-3 fatty acids in your supplement, you'll want to check the ingredient label to ensure at least 1,000 mg of EPA and/or DHA are indicated, which equates to one gram of these fatty acids. While 1,000 mg of omega-3s is the minimum dosage, increasing the dosage to 3,000 mg daily can also be therapeutic for supporting endocrine function and lowering inflammation systemically.[19]

Supplementation with omega-3 fatty acids during pregnancy lowers the risk of premature birth and can increase the length of pregnancy and birth weight by altering the balance of eicosanoids involved in labor and promote fetal growth by improving placental blood flow.[20] Intake of omega-3 fatty acids during pregnancy and breast feeding may facilitate the child's brain development, and evidence suggests that they prevent preeclampsia, postpartum depression, menopausal problems, postmenopausal osteoporosis, and breast cancer.[21] Needless to say, omega-3 is something that is helpful to consume during pregnancy, and starting in the preconception phase cannot only help hormone production for conception, but can also facilitate hormone levels through childbirth and postpartum, in addition to supporting healthy fetal development.

Of note, EPA and DHA are essential for neurological development of children in utero, and a minimum of 2,000 mg in the first half of pregnancy, and 4,000 mg in the second half of pregnancy, are advised. Without adequate dietary intake, you'll be further depleted in your efforts to give everything to your baby for healthy development.

Fat-soluble vitamins (ADEK)

Deficiencies in fat-soluble vitamins (vitamins A, D, E, and K) are a core issue in infertility and support for conception, as they're essential for fetal growth and development.[22]

Vitamin A (retinol) assists the follicles in the maturation of the egg and helps to produce hormones needed to aid the fertilized egg into the uterus.[23] Vitamin A also supports both male and female reproduction as well as embryonic development.[24]

Studies show that women that meet the requirements for vitamin D levels in blood serum are more likely to conceive[25] and that low vitamin D status is a factor in infertility as a whole, with supplementation showing improved pregnancy outcomes.[26] Vitamin D also supports immune function, which is what it is most commonly associated with, and as such, supports the healthy prevention of internal pathogens. When vitamin D levels are low, it's helpful to consider if consumption, synthesis, or uses are depleting levels and to address food, supplementation, healthy synthesis, and reducing infections in the body, such as gut pathogens.

While supplementing with vitamin D, retinol, and other fat-soluble vitamins can be helpful, it's not always the best or most effective option. Since these are fat-soluble, you'll often see them encapsulated alongside a carrier oil to promote absorption. However, if fat digestion and absorption are impaired due to poor bile production, gallbladder dysfunction, or impaired fat absorption, (as we discussed in Chapter 13) the absorption of fat-soluble vitamins will also be impacted. Therefore, the first step in ensuring adequate fat-soluble vitamins is to support the digestion of fats themselves through liver support and digestion function.

According to the Food and Nutrition Board (FNB), which determines recommended daily allowances, women need 700 mcg daily of retinol. However, retinol intake needs are typically based on thyroid function, with higher thyroid function requiring more. Morley Robbins suggests that the proper ratio of vitamin A to vitamin D is 10:1, which is why supplementing with vitamin D is not always helpful and can throw off the balance between all fat-soluble vitamins.[27]

Vitamin D is also synthesized in the body, particularly through activation in the skin in response to UVB exposure (i.e., sunshine). Since vitamin D is present in very few foods, unprotected sun exposure is the best way to support healthy vitamin D levels. This means that skin is exposed without sunscreen or other sun protection.

Regardless of the source of vitamin D, when it enters the body, it's in a biologically inert form that requires two phases of chemical processes to be converted into its active form, calcitriol, which is a steroid hormone. The first chemical process occurs in the liver to convert vitamin D to 25-hydroxy vitamin D [25(OH)D], also known as calcidiol, while the second process occurs in the kidneys to form the physiologically active 1,25-dihydroxy vitamin D [1,25(OH)2D] - also known as calcitriol. As such, the health of these organs is important in supporting healthy vitamin D levels.

One of the best food sources for both retinol and vitamin D is cod liver oil, as it contains 4,500 IU of vitamin A and 450 IU of vitamin D per teaspoon.[28] Note that cod liver oil contains these vitamins, but may be lacking in adequate EPA and DHA, which means supplementation of both may be warranted. While this might not be enough to support vitamin D needs daily, cod liver oil is one of the only food sources that contains vitamin D. Other foods that are robust sources of retinol include turkey, and liver from beef, chicken, and pork, as well as butter, ghee, egg yolks, raw cheeses, and milks.

The therapeutic dosage of vitamin D in supplement form will depend on the severity of the deficiency, but typically, 5,000 IU daily is recommended when using a carrier fat. Testing for serum vitamin D is essential for determining true nutritional needs, with below 40 ng/ml being suboptimal levels of serum vitamin D.[29]

Choline

Choline is an essential nutrient naturally present in foods such as liver, egg yolks, and red meat. It's a source of methyl groups needed for many steps in the process of methylation in the liver. The body needs choline to synthesize phosphatidylcholine and sphingomyelin, two major phospholipids vital for the health of cell membranes, and it is required by all plant and animal cells to preserve their structural integrity.[30]

Choline is also needed for the production of neurotransmitters and other brain and nervous system functions, and plays a role in modulating gene expression, cell membrane signaling, and lipid metabolism.[31]

Choline is an underrecognized nutrient needed for the support of conception, as well as throughout pregnancy. Not only does choline help support healthy ovarian function, but improved pregnancy outcomes are associated with choline supplementation.[32] It also increases the percentage of antral follicles, and increases levels and interactions of hormone receptors for vital hormones including luteinizing hormone.[33] Found in large amounts in the placenta, amniotic fluid, and breast milk, choline is recommended in a dosage of 450 mg per day.

Fetal brain development, gene expression, membrane biosynthesis, and tissue expansion are all important prenatal processes that require ample choline levels in the maternal diet.[34] Studies have shown that supplementing the diet with choline improves pregnancy outcomes and reduces the risk of negative outcomes, such as neural tube defects and preeclampsia.[35]

Unfortunately, most prenatal vitamins do not contain choline, or if they do, it's at minimal levels. Why is this? Choline is a bulky nutrient and requires a large amount of space in the capsule of prenatal vitamins, which often requires consumption of several capsules in order to achieve the recommended dosage. It's also not the most affordable nutrient, and as such, many prenatal vitamins choose to exclude it from their formulation. If you're currently taking a prenatal vitamin in preparation for pregnancy, it's a good thing to check the nutrition facts and either switch to a prenatal vitamin containing choline or consider adding one to your existing regime.

If there is not an adequate amount of choline in the body, the maternal plasma choline can become depleted.[36] Keep in mind that the time period following a miscarriage is considered postpartum and can contribute to depletions of choline, so this is worth considering if you have experienced one or more miscarriages.

Iron

Iron anemia has been related to infertility, miscarriage, and poor pregnancy outcomes,[37] and adequate iron is a crucial factor for supporting conception, but it doesn't always mean that supplementing with iron is needed or recommended. Ferritin is also not the best indicator of iron deficiency, since it represents the stored form of iron in the liver rather than available iron in the blood serum.[38] Total serum iron alongside ferritin can more accurately provide a depiction of iron availability and absorption in the body.

First, let's consider where we get iron from in the diet. There are two forms of iron: heme iron and non-heme iron. Heme iron comes from animal sources and is the most bioavailable form of iron, with a 10% iron availability rate. Non-heme iron on the other hand comes from plant-based sources, which is an inferior source of iron and only 1% absorbable.[39] This is one of many reasons that animal protein is essential for healthy conception and pregnancies.[40]

So if you're already eating animal proteins and still have iron anemia, next you'll want to consider if you're chemically able to break down the foods that contain iron to ensure absorption of this mineral. We covered this in depth in the Chapter 13, but suffice it to say that optimizing and supporting hydrochloric acid (HCl) levels in the stomach are essential in resolving iron anemia.[41] It's for this reason that those with low HCl, H. pylori infections, and the presence of upper gastrointestinal symptoms often struggle with iron anemia.

You can also support the absorption of iron while reducing the inhibition of absorption through the food you eat. Vitamin C plays a crucial role in the absorption of iron, so consuming plenty of vitamin C-rich foods like berries, citrus fruits, bell peppers, and potatoes helps promote the absorption of iron, especially when consumed alongside iron-rich foods. Think steak and potatoes. You can also supplement with Vitamin C, in which case a daily dose of 250 mg of vitamin C (taken with iron-rich meals) is a good general guideline.[42]

Other foods can impair the absorption of iron, such as tea, coffee, dairy, supplementation fiber, and supplements with calcium or zinc in them.[43] These foods don't need to be completely avoided, but it's advisable to keep them away from the iron-rich foods you intend to absorb.

If iron anemia still persists, you'll want to consider the fact that all organisms utilize iron to survive, and pathogens in the gut may be stealing this nutrient from you, creating a blocking factor for fertility.[44] While parasites are the most likely culprit, addressing your unique microbiome to restore balance and ensure you're the one reaping the benefits of your nutrient-dense diet will assist in resolving iron deficiencies.

Only in very rare circumstances is it advised to utilize an iron supplement to restore iron levels in the body. When ferritin is the only iron marker that is low, supplementing with iron can actually cause more harm than good. In fact, ferritin is formed in the gut lining, so supporting digestion will typically help dramatically improve this marker. Iron is oxidative in the body, which means it can "rust" and cause cellular damage and an increase in free radicals.[45] If iron is not truly low, and only ferritin is depressed, this oxidative cellular damage can cause even further damage and make matters worse, without managing to support low ferritin at all.

Starting with animal protein sources, supporting digestion and absorption while being mindful of absorption-impairing foods can help bring iron back into balance and promote a healthy pregnancy from the time of conception all the way through birth.

Glycine

Given that nearly all of us are subjected to small doses of glyphosate in our lives -whether through our food, the air we breathe, or the environments that we frequent - supporting the damaging effects of glyphosate is a crucial part of supporting nutritional deficiencies for fertility.

As we have discussed in depth, one of the key nutrients depleted by glyphosate is glycine, due to its similar biochemical structure. This amino acid is crucial for several processes in the body and can be acquired through supplementation or food. As such, supplementation with glycine and consuming glycine-rich foods are a great way to ensure deficiencies are restored and that the inevitable harms of glyphosate exposure are minimized. Food sources of glycine include animal proteins, salmon, peanuts, and bone broth. For supplementation, you might consider collagen and full amino acid supplements to maintain the balance of all amino acids. Of note, glycine is synthesized in our body from choline as well.

Chapter 16
Dietary Strategies for Hormone Health

CORE PRINCIPLE NINE: Nourish yourself with whole, nutrient-dense foods that promote healthy inflammation levels.

In addition to ensuring the high quality of the food you consume, you can do so much with dietary changes to support conception and healthy hormones. In addition to a nutrient-dense diet, there are several strategies to consider to support healthy blood sugar regulation. The food you eat nourishes you or slowly contributes to the decline of your health, and many of the decisions we make affecting our longevity and the health of our children (and grandchildren) begin on our very own dinner plate.

General guidelines

A lot of dogma and confusion around nutrition exists in our world today. From extreme diets that remove an entire macronutrient (like carbs in the ketogenic diet or protein in vegan diets), everyone is looking for the best way to eat to support their health goals. With fertility and healthy hormones in mind, there are some specific guidelines we'll discuss, but I want to emphasize that there are only a few important things that matter. So much of nutrition is truly bioindividual and what works best for me may very likely not work well for you. We're different people, obviously. While there may be some important considerations to ensure you have the necessary building blocks to facilitate healthy hormones, you won't find any extreme nutrition dogma here.

What I've seen is that most of us typically already know what is best for us. You know what foods work for you and what foods don't, and while I certainly want to make some key recommendations, I don't think you need to be fearful of carbs, sugar, or red meat. Most of us who are health conscious are already doing a pretty good job of nourishing our body, even when our diet is not perfect.

Food quality over everything

To put it simply, a whole food, nutrient-dense diet is going to serve you best throughout your fertility journey, as well as through pregnancy, and it sets the stage to raise healthy children as well. This means that processed foods are minimized, but also with some realism. We can't all eat fresh produce with locally raised protein at every meal. Sometimes, we need to lean on a frozen meal or a bag of chips, and turn to something that is processed so that it keeps well while traveling.

If you're not familiar with Weston A. Price's work, here's the background. Price was a dentist who traveled the world in the 1930s to observe the facial structures of people with varying diets, with the goal of discovering which factors contributed to good oral health. His studies revealed that dental caries and deformed dental arches resulting in crowded, crooked teeth are the result of nutritional deficiencies, not inherited genetic defects.[1] He found that in isolated communities where people consumed large quantities of fats and fat-soluble vitamins, they not only had better oral health but also understood the importance of preconception nutrition for both partners. Many tribes honored a period of "special feeding" before conception, in which nutrient-dense animal foods were given to young men and women, which contributed to an ease of reproduction, emotional stability, and freedom from degenerative illnesses, especially when compared to civilized modern societies consuming more sugar, white flour, pasteurized milk, low-fat foods, vegetable oils, and convenience items filled with extenders and additives.

As a result of his work traveling for nearly a decade, Price formulated the following principles[2] for dietary guidelines:

1. Eat whole, unprocessed foods.
2. Eat beef, lamb, game, organ meats, poultry, and eggs from pasture-fed animals.

3. Eat wild fish (not farm-raised), fish eggs, and shellfish from unpolluted waters.
4. Eat full-fat milk products from pasture-fed cows, preferably raw and/or fermented, such as raw milk, whole yogurt, kefir, cultured butter, full-fat raw cheeses, and fresh and sour cream.
5. Use animal fats, such as lard, tallow, egg yolks, cream, and butter, liberally.
6. Use only traditional vegetable oils (such as extra virgin olive oil, expeller-expressed sesame oil, small amounts of expeller-expressed flax oil, and the tropical oils), coconut oil, palm oil, and palm kernel oil.
7. Take cod liver oil regularly to provide at least 10,000 IU vitamin A and 1,000 IU vitamin D per day.
8. Eat fresh fruits and vegetables, preferably organic. Use vegetables in salads and soups, or lightly steamed with butter.
9. Use organic whole grains, legumes, and nuts that have been prepared by soaking, sprouting, or sour leavening to neutralize phytic acid, enzyme inhibitors, and other anti-nutrients.
10. Include enzyme-rich lacto-fermented vegetables, fruits, beverages, and condiments in your diet on a regular basis (kimchi, kefir, sauerkraut, etc.).
11. Prepare homemade stocks from the bones of pastured poultry, beef, pork, and lamb, and from wild seafood. Use liberally in soups, stews, gravies, and sauces.
12. Use filtered water for cooking and drinking.
13. Use unrefined salt and a variety of herbs and spices for food interest and appetite stimulation.
14. Make your own salad dressing using raw vinegar, extra virgin olive oil, and a small amount of expeller-pressed flax oil.
15. Use traditional sweeteners in moderation, such as raw honey, maple syrup, maple sugar, date sugar, and green stevia powder.
16. Use only unpasteurized wine or beer in strict moderation with meals.

These guidelines can seem very strict, and as I mentioned, I don't necessarily recommend living and breathing by these recommendations, but aiming for these and implementing as many of these recommendations as frequently as possible promotes vitality in the preconception and conception seasons of life.

Important notes on these recommendations

Animal protein is essential for conception and pregnancy. Protein is quite literally the building block for all human life, with every cell in your body containing amino acids that are needed to build new cells, which you can imagine is a huge goal of pregnancy, as we literally build a baby from scratch. Without adequate intake of amino acids and proteins, your body will ultimately pull these essential amino acids from your body, depleting you, in the process of supporting a healthy baby in utero. However, if it's unable to do this due to low protein intake, impaired digestion, or poor reserves to utilize in your body, cell division in the fetus can struggle to occur at necessary rates.

Animal proteins are complete proteins, meaning they contain all of the essential amino acids you need when compared to plant-proteins, which contain less of these amino acids, as well as far less nutrients and calories. Furthermore, animal proteins are a more efficient delivery system and are easier for us to digest, and therefore, to benefit from.

In *Real Food for Pregnancy*, Lily Nichols outlines protein needs during pregnancy, which serve as a good starting point for protein intake in the preconception phase as well. In a study conducted in 2015, women's protein needs were found to be 39% higher in early pregnancy and 73% higher in late pregnancy, compared to the estimated average requirement.[3] They found that the guideline for protein needs in early pregnancy is 1.22g/kg and 1.52 g/kg in late pregnancy. Nutrient requirements are calculated based on a woman's pre-pregnancy weight; this means a woman who started her pregnancy at 150 pounds would need 83 g of protein in early pregnancy and 104 g of protein/day in late pregnancy.

For individuals with severely protein-deficient states, compromised ability to break down protein, and for those who have used a vegan or vegetarian diet in the past, recommendations may need to be much higher in a healing phase. As such, my recommendations for protein consumption typically fall between 100–150 grams of protein per day based on your height, weight, physical activity, and satiety. Remember, you are uniquely you, so you might find that you actually feel better with more protein in your diet.

Vegetable and canola oils

If there is just one thing you should get rid of in your diet, particularly when cooking at home, it's hydrogenated, refined cooking oil (i.e., vegetable and canola oil). It's the only thing that I routinely tell clients to throw away and never buy again, not for cooking your dinner, not for baking, not for anything. This speaks directly to how toxic these cooking oils are for us.

These oils have become the preferred oils used by food industries, and fast food and regular restaurants, because they are extremely cheap and can keep their food shelf-stable for an extremely long time. But this shelf-stability comes at the cost of high calories, while being low in nutrition, containing chemical residues and trans fats (well-documented in contributing to cardiovascular disease), and are highly oxidized, resulting in damaged molecules that cause inflammation and irritation systemically once consumed.

Throw them out if they are still in your kitchen, and check ingredient labels of any processed foods (think packaged, not fresh), to see if they include vegetable or canola oil and make healthier swaps when possible. Fortunately, many alternatives do now exist that utilize more stable cooking fats such as avocado and coconut oil.

Salt

Salt and sodium have gotten a bad reputation and have become the scapegoat for many of the things that added sugars have done to our health over the last several decades. Many people have become fearful of sodium in relation to blood pressure.

In *The Salt Fix*, Dr. James DiNicolantonio's research shows that the optimal salt intake is around 3,000–5,000 mg of sodium per day for most people. This is significantly higher than the 2,300 mg that Americans are cautioned against exceeding on a daily basis. Sodium isn't the only factor here, and as with most things, quality matters.

Iodized salt is not something you'll want to consume in large quantities, as it is lacking the electrolytes and minerals that assist in balancing the sodium for healthy use in the body. Instead, unrefined salts are best: Himalayan, Celtic, Redmond Real Salt, and other unrefined options not only provide sodium that is derived from evaporated seawater to extract natural salts, but also contain dozens of other minerals, such as potassium, to not only balance the sodium, but nourish you deeply.

Not only can these salts be used to season your food sparingly, but adding salt to water can also assist in hydration.

Calorie intake

Are you eating enough? Probably not.

Did you know that toddlers require 1,200 calories per day to support the size of their bodies? So why is 1,200 the number of calories women often refer to as an upper caloric limit on a daily basis, so they can maintain their figure and promote health? This low-calorie goal is especially not supportive of trying to conceive, nor does it support the integral work the must occur to support ovulation, healthy hormones, egg fertilization, and the replication of cells that happens at miraculous speeds in early pregnancy.

You need to be eating at least 2,000 calories a day.

If that number scares you, and you're concerned I'm trying to make you gain weight, I can tell you that research shows that grown women need this many calories to support all of the functions in the body.

To give you another reference point, your basal metabolic rate (BMR) is something you can calculate. Your BMR is calculated based on your height, weight, and age to determine the daily caloric needs to support your body at full rest. This means that the BMR is indicative of the amount of calories you need to be consuming on a daily basis if you were to simply lie in bed all day, and just be alive.

Figure 16.1

WOMEN

$$\textbf{BMR} = (10 \times \text{weight [kg]}) + (6.25 \times \text{heigh[cm]}) - (5 \times \text{age [yrs]}) - 161$$

Often when calculating your own BMR, you'll find that you are drastically undereating even to meet the baseline caloric needs to support organ function, let alone the exercise, work stress, and movement that you experience on a daily basis. From your BMR, you need to also increase calorie intake to support physical activity frequency. For instance, if you are working out five days per week, you need to increase the caloric intake calculated from your BMR by roughly 500 calories for every single day.

You may need to increase your caloric intake slowly over several weeks and track your caloric intake, as well as your protein intake, in particular. Free tracking apps, such as My Fitness Pal and Cronometer, are available to help you do this. This kind of tracking can be an eye-opening exercise to better support nourishing your body for fertility, in addition to sharpening your focus on food quality.

Fats (and cholesterol) are your friend

As you can see in Figure 16.2, all steroid hormones are derived from cholesterol. Cholesterol is used to develop pregnenolone, often referred to as the "mother hormone," given its role in the production of all hormones in the ovaries and adrenals that play a crucial role in fertility.

Progesterone deficiency is a common occurrence with fertility concerns, and as you can see, progesterone cannot be produced without adequate pregnenolone and therefore, cholesterol. Given cholesterol's prominent position at the top of the steroid hormone pathway, it is easy to see how a low-fat diet can lead to hormonal imbalances downstream.

Figure 16.2

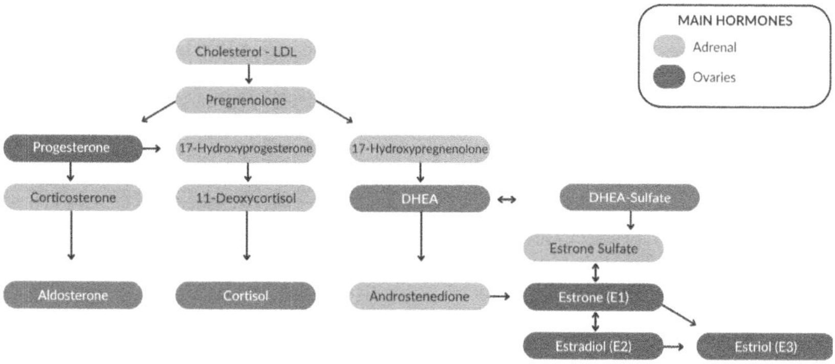

Hydration

In addition to food quality and types, hydration is particularly important for the health of the body, and all systems rely on adequate hydration to function optimally. This means that adequate water intake is an important factor. Unfortunately, much of the advice around water intake is convoluted and not based on research, nor does it support cellular hydration.

Ideally, you're consuming around half of your body weight in ounces of water daily. For example, if you weigh 150 pounds, you should be consuming around 75 ounces of water daily, not to include any caffeinated beverages. You'll notice that this is much less than the recommended gallon of water typically recommended for hydration. There's such a thing as too much water and over-hydrating cells, but it's more likely that you're simply flushing your system rather than absorbing any water for use at such high intake levels.

In addition to quantity, using electrolytes to support cellular hydration is crucial and something that most people are missing. While we commonly think of electrolytes as minerals that support the absorption of water at a cellular level, electrolytes are minerals that have a positive or negative charge when dissolved in water, body fluids, or blood. These electrical charges facilitate the movement of water into and out of different tissues and cells, as well as balance pH level in the body, regulate blood pressure, and support the communication between all cells.[4] At our core, we are electric beings, and we need electricity charges to communicate between our cells. Electrolytes support these mechanisms to support optimal organ function.

Regardless of the type of water you're drinking, minerals and electrolytes should be utilized daily to support the absorption of water. Remember that if you're drinking reverse osmosis or distilled water as recommended, you must replenish minerals in your water. A pinch of salt water with lemon juice can be used to support cellular hydration, or you can add a higher-dose sodium electrolyte additive to water.

Adding humic and fulvic acid to your water source is another way to not only support hydration, but to also support natural detoxification from industrial chemicals like glyphosate and promote the absorption of water-soluble nutrients. Humic and fulvic acids are composed of materials from the Earth's natural materials, including the ocean, woods, compost piles, and even our gardens. These potent nutrients are supportive of our health through the innate wisdom of the Earth and the natural cycle of materials that break down over time.

Blood sugar regulation

While you might normally think of blood sugar dysregulation as diabetes, there is a much wider spectrum for blood sugar concerns that impact hypothalamic-pituitary (HP) function. HP function is responsible for the orchestration of all endocrine glands in the body, which means that if you have hormonal irregularities, you must consider blood sugar dysregulation. It's not enough to say, "I eat clean, I eat well, and there's no way that blood sugar is an issue."

Most women who eat quality produce and meats and are mindful of both sugar and processed carbohydrate intake still have blood sugar dysregulation. In fact, if you're reading this and don't think blood sugar is a concern for you, bless you – because it's a concern for all of us to varying degrees of severity. I'm not knocking you, but our culture is not designed to support blood sugar regulation. Consider the typical day of our modern lives: We are wakened by an alarm, out of alignment with our circadian rhythms, drink coffee on an empty stomach to further wake up, and often skip breakfast. Throughout the day, we eat a low-calorie and low-fat diet, even limiting carbs because we fear them, go long stretches between meals, live stressful lives in front of screens, and deprive ourselves of the required 7–8 hours of sleep we need daily. We can see that food is not the only thing disrupting our ability to have picture-perfect blood sugar regulation, nor is perfection the goal.

Blood sugar is a crucial component of all hormone health, because as we've discussed, hormones do not function in a bubble and blood glucose is regulated by a series of hormonal interactions to maintain glucose stability. For example, when blood glucose levels drop, the body responds by releasing cortisol to bring glucose levels back into a normal healthy level. While we are asleep, the adrenals release adrenaline in response to blood sugar crashing, which typically results in waking in the middle of the night. This release of cortisol can suppress the production of sex hormones such as testosterone and estrogen, leading to imbalances.[5] Low blood sugar can also impact levels of insulin, which plays a role in regulating the production and release of sex hormones from the ovaries,[6] meaning that low insulin levels can lead to decreased production of estrogen, resulting in menstrual irregularities or even amenorrhea (absence of menstruation).[7]

Now imagine if this is happening multiple times per day due to consuming high carbohydrate meals, or even just meals that are spiking blood sugar, and therefore causing a blood sugar crash in the hours after a meal.

Figure 16.3

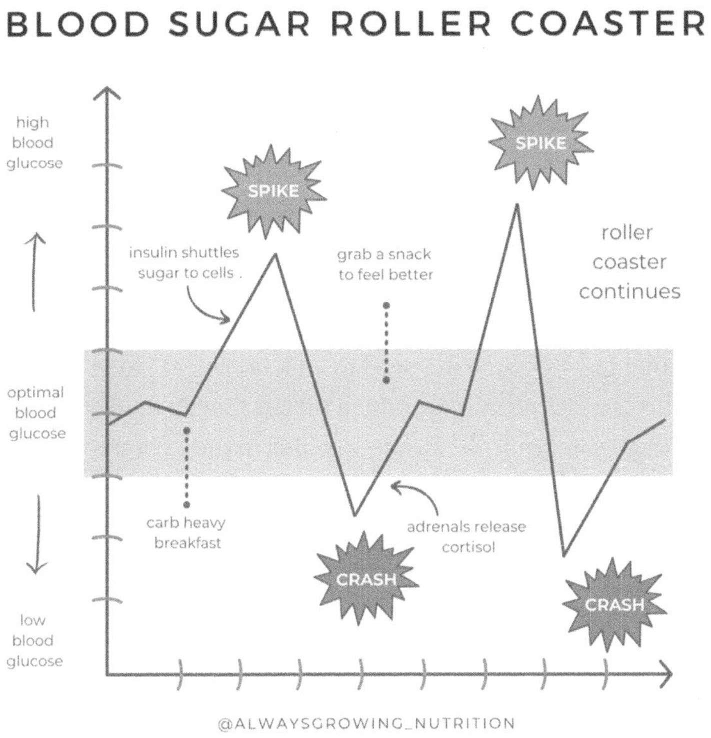

Getting to know your blood sugar

First, it can be helpful to assess your blood sugar situation. Bloodwork tells us a lot about the clinical picture of blood sugar management, as do our symptoms.

Hemoglobin A1c is conventionally used in the screening and diagnosis of diabetes and other blood sugar-related diseases. This marker provides a retrospective look at blood sugar handling, as it looks at the average glucose over the prior 120 days by looking at the red blood cells. The normal lifespan of a red blood cell is 120 days, and glucose combines with hemoglobin to produce "glycohemoglobin." The amount of glycohemoglobin formed is reflective of the amount of glucose present in the bloodstream during the 120 days of that red blood cell's lifespan. Higher levels of glycohemoglobin indicate more glucose was present in the blood during those 120 days, while lower levels of glycohemoglobin indicate less glucose was present during those 120 days.

This allows you to look back and get the "average" glucose in the bloodstream that has interacted with red blood cells during that time. While the conventional range for HbA1c is 4.1–5.7%, functional range is 4.1–5.4%.

For a look at current blood glucose levels, blood measures can also be taken at any time to determine the amount of glucose present in the bloodstream. Fasting glucose is a true snapshot in time and can be a good marker to determine the need to look further at blood sugar regulation. This is a fasting marker, which means that all food and beverages other than water must be strictly avoided in the 12 hours prior to the test, in order to determine how the body is able to manage blood sugar in the absence of all food. Fasting glucose should optimally be between 70–90 mg/dL, and when your fasting levels are outside of this range, it can begin to give you clues about potential hyperglycemia or (more commonly) hypoglycemia.

Testing your blood glucose at home is not only incredibly easy, but incredibly affordable. While you can certainly have a blood draw at a lab to determine your fasting glucose levels first thing in the morning, you can also obtain information at home using a finger-prick glucose monitor. While fasting glucose is often representative of the whole day, you can also look deeper at glucose following meals (also known as postprandial measurements). Postprandial glucose levels are expected to be higher in response to any meal, regardless of carbohydrate content, and will decline slowly in the hours following a meal, ideally landing back at your fasting glucose level within four hours. Looking at postprandial blood sugar can also provide valuable insight about what meals are working well for you, as well as specific foods and quantities of foods that negatively affect blood sugar, causing a spike (and a resulting a crash).

Ideally, postprandial levels should fall within these limits:

- Fasting glucose: 70–90 mg/dL
- 1-hour postprandial: 100–130 mg/dL
- 2-hours postprandial: 100–120 mg/dL
- 3-hours postprandial: 90–110 mg/dL
- 4-hours postprandial: 70–90 mg/dL

If pricking your finger several times per day for multiple days sounds like torture, you might instead consider a continuous glucose monitor (CGM), which is applied on the back of your arm with a sensor and electrode that remains in the skin to detect changes in blood sugar for up to two weeks per sensor. These devices connect to your phone to sync data automatically, which allows you to review the information, observe glucose spikes and crashes, record your meals, and formulate changes to better support reducing the curve of your blood sugar. These CGMs are becoming more readily available, but you do require a prescription to access them. Your primary care physician can prescribe one for you to go through insurance, or you can get help obtaining one in the Resources at the end of this book.

Insulin is another marker done via blood draw that can provide insight into your blood sugar regulation, particularly if insulin resistance is suspected. Insulin itself is a hormone and its primary role is the shuttling of glucose to cells for use. It does this by binding to receptor sites on cells to indicate the need to absorb glucose for energy. The optimal range for fasting insulin is 2–8 μU/ml, which is significantly different than conventional ranges. Keep in mind that while insulin is conventionally used to diagnose for insulinoma (insulin-producing pancreatic islet cell tumors), the functional range is where things should be optimally in healthy blood sugar management.

Elevated insulin is typically caused by insulin resistance, where the pancreas is secreting high amounts of insulin to keep up with glucose levels, but the cell receptors are desensitized to it, thus creating a vicious cycle where even more insulin is secreted in an attempt to communicate with the cells. We'll discuss the role of insulin sensitivity in the progression of blood sugar issues, shortly.

On the other hand, when insulin is low, it can be indicative of excess blood glucose, hyperglycemia, diabetes, hypopituitarism, or some form of pancreatic disease.

The last marker to assist in your understanding of your blood sugar management is lactate dehydrogenase (LDH). This is an enzyme that supports the conversion of pyruvate to lactate. Pyruvate is the final product of glycolysis, and it's converted to lactate when oxygen is absent or in short supply. It also reverses this mechanism by anaerobic glycolysis in the muscles, and then moves to the liver and is converted to glucose to be released back into the bloodstream. Suboptimal LDH tells us more about blood sugar regulation, as the body attempts to release converted glucose into the bloodstream to maintain and uplift glucose levels. Low levels indicate that the body is lacking in adequate glucose to feed the biochemical process that produces ATP, often due to hypoglycemia. LDH can also be low in a case of insulin resistance. If cells aren't accepting glucose, they don't need pyruvate to make energy; therefore, the LDH activity ramps down.

Hypoglycemia (or low blood glucose) is so common, it's considered normal. Have you ever used the term "hangry" when you're starving and feel better after eating? That's hypoglycemia, and it looks different from person to person but is generally accepted as a normal human condition. Just because it's common doesn't mean it's normal, and it's a sign of poor sugar handling.

Symptoms that commonly indicate hypoglycemia:

- Shaky or lightheaded if meals are skipped (or delayed)
- A craving for sweets or carbohydrates of any kind (including alcohol, fruit and starchy foods). This usually happens after meals (e.g., always needing a dessert) or late in the evening.
- Headaches and migraines
- Irritability before meals (i.e., getting "hangry")
- Sleep disruptions: difficulty falling asleep, staying asleep (waking between 1 and 4 a.m.), and waking at night to urinate
- Needing coffee to function in the morning (or late afternoon)
- Episodes of depression, anxiety, irritability, and mood swings
- Brain fog or an inability to think clearly
- Fatigue that is relieved by eating

There are two types of hypoglycemia: – fasting hypoglycemia and reactive hypoglycemia. While the symptoms are often the same, the approach for resolution can vary. Suboptimal LDH is often more indicative of reactive hypoglycemia, often in part due to long stretches of time between meals.

On the opposite end of the spectrum is hyperglycemia, or elevated glucose levels.

Symptoms commonly associated with hyperglycemia include:

- Poor wound healing
- Frequent thirst and urination
- Excessive hunger
- Eye issues (blurry vision, cataracts, glaucoma, and retinopathy)
- Poor circulation (cold hands and feet)
- Stomach aches

- Feeling wired, then tired
- Puffiness and inflammation
- Acne
- Headaches
- Recurrent infections (skin, yeast, bladder)
- Neuropathy (tingling hands and feet)
- Skin tags

Chronic elevated glucose levels alter metabolism and contribute to cardiovascular disease, sleep apnea, hormone imbalances, and obesity.

When insulin is elevated, oxidative stress increases free radical production, speeding up the aging process. Blood pressure increases in response to the demands put on the adrenal glands, which are responsible for the regulation of blood pressure. Lipogenesis and cholesterol synthesis are increased, often resulting in elevated cholesterol levels. Elevated insulin also interferes with adrenal and sex hormones. For women, elevated insulin increases the production of testosterone, while for men it increases the conversion of testosterone to estrogen. Excess insulin has also been linked to the promotion of carcinogenesis and thus, an increased risk of some cancers.

To illustrate the importance of blood sugar regardless of a hypo- or hyperglycemia presentation, it can be helpful to understand how blood sugar issues progress over time. As hypoglycemia is very common, this is typically where things start, whether it's fasting hypoglycemia or being reactive to meals. The drops of blood glucose often occur in response to a meal and an insulin spike in the attempt to shuttle glucose to cells for use. Over time, high insulin spikes can create a desensitization of insulin at the level of cell receptors, contributing to insulin resistance.

Insulin resistance is a complex metabolic condition resulting from multiple contributing factors, including a diet high in refined carbohydrates, a lifestyle lacking in physical activity, excess weight, and hormonal imbalances. While it can take a long time for insulin resistance to progress, it can ultimately result in diabetes, where the body is unable to keep up with insulin demands and requires exogenous support (i.e. must take insulin). Metabolic syndrome is the next phase of blood sugar dysregulation. It's a collection of symptoms, including insulin resistance, that drastically increases the likelihood of cardiovascular disease involvement and is categorized by elevated triglycerides, elevated total cholesterol levels, low HDL (good cholesterol), increased blood pressure, and often, obesity. Sound familiar here in the United States?

Tackling blood sugar problems

Whether the issue is hypoglycemia or hyperglycemia, you'll want to start by focusing on food quality, as well as a number of dietary and lifestyle strategies to support healthy blood sugar levels, and therefore, "happy" hormones as a whole.

Blood sugar can be negatively affected by toxin burden. Cellular health is impacted by toxins, illness, and other environmental factors that can contribute to inflammation and impact cell signaling. For instance, PCBs, BPA, arsenic, phthalates, perfluorinates (PFOS), diethyl hexyl phthalate (DEHP), and dioxin (TCDD) all negatively impact blood sugar regulation.[8] This is yet another way that lowering toxin exposure is crucial for supporting your health.

To balance blood sugar naturally and ensure variety in the diet, we ideally want there to be 3 things in each meal: protein, fat, and fiber. Protein is going to primarily consist of animal proteins and byproducts (such as eggs and milk), which helps to keep you full and satiated between meals, while also ensuring that your body is not breaking down muscle mass for fuel. Protein is the number-one thing to help support the stabilization of blood sugar at each meal. Ideally you're consuming 4–6 ounces of animal meat, 3–4 whole eggs, or a protein powder, all of which should equate to a minimum of 30 grams of protein per meal. As a trick, your protein portion at each meal should be roughly the size of your palm – both as big as the surface area and as thick.

Healthy dietary fats are next, as these are not only necessary for cellular hormone sensitivity, cell membrane structure, and hormone production, but they also significantly slow the digestion of sugar to stabilize blood sugar. Instead of getting a dramatic spike in blood sugar, the inclusion of healthy fats with meals helps to promote a gentle wave of glucose increasing. Aim for around 1–2 tablespoons of fat per meal, whether this is in the form of your cooking oil or in a high-fat protein, egg yolks, avocados, nuts, or seeds. As a trick, this portion should be roughly the size of two of your thumbs, (where 1 thumb equates to 1 tablespoon).

Last is fiber, which is primarily found in carbohydrates. Remember that carbohydrates are not the enemy, but we want to be mindful of processed carbohydrates and those containing added sugars. If we think of sugar as "poison," think about fiber as the antidote. Fiber is found in fruits and vegetables, which naturally contain sugars, and yet, these types of foods do not spike blood glucose the same way that cane sugar, breads, and pastas do. This is because fiber slows the speed in which glucose is absorbed. To support healthy fiber intake, aim for 4–7 non-starchy, whole vegetable servings per day, 1–3 whole fruit servings per day, and 1–3 starchy carbohydrate sources (potatoes, winter squashes, beans, legumes/peas, rice, etc.) per day. As a trick when you can't measure, vegetable intake should be around 1–2 cups or 1-2 fist-sized portions per meal, while fruit and starchy carbs should be around a half a cup or a cupped handful portion per meal.

In addition to minimizing the consumption of processed carbohydrates and sugary foods, you'll also want to ensure you aren't eating "naked carbs." This term refers to any meal or snack where only carbohydrates are being consumed. For example, oatmeal for breakfast contains only carbohydrates, and these "naked carbs" will inevitably cause a spike in blood glucose followed by a crash. By adding protein and fats to these meals, you'll notice significant improvements in blood sugar handling, without removing the carbohydrate altogether. The work of Jessie Inchauspé in the book, *Glucose Revolution: The Life-Changing Power of*

Balancing Your Blood Sugar, perfectly illustrates several scenarios where the addition of proteins, carbs, and even fiber to meals dramatically shifts the response in blood glucose.

Breakfast sets the tone for blood sugar for the day. If the first meal of the day triggers a blood glucose spike and crash, it's nearly impossible to restore balance and stop the progression of the blood sugar roller coaster throughout the day. As such, focusing on your first meal of the day is crucial for setting the stage for blood sugar stability. When designing this meal, most women feel best when consuming primarily protein and fat with minimal carbohydrates, but you should find what works best for you. It's also crucial to eat within 30 minutes of waking (rather than waiting several hours), which will help promote a healthy metabolism. This timing also reduces stress hormones (cortisol) in the morning to further support hormone balance.

Coffee should always be had alongside or after breakfast, but never on an empty stomach. The caffeine in coffee increases cortisol levels in the body, but can result in blood sugar dysregulation, which is not seen when caffeine is consumed with food. This will also help encourage you to eat shortly after waking.

Meal sequencing is another strategy scientifically proven to support better blood sugar regulation. This strategy looks at the order in which you eat the foods on your plate and how this impacts blood glucose response, for better or for worse. Eating fiber-rich foods before consuming proteins and fats, and leaving starchy carbohydrates for last, drastically reduces blood sugar spikes.

Next, consider the timing of your meals throughout the day. If you're struggling with hypoglycemia, it's crucial to ensure you aren't skipping meals and are eating every 2–3 hours to keep blood glucose within optimal ranges. Once your blood glucose levels have evened out and you are no longer experiencing a glucose crash, you can stretch the time between meals to 4–5 hours, but the gap shouldn't be longer than this benchmark. This might mean that you need to have an additional meal or snack during the day, which is okay.

Certain types of foods are also supportive of healthy blood sugar and can be incorporated into your diet. Bitter foods, such as arugula, endive, radicchio, mustard greens, and dandelion greens stimulate liver function, which is crucial for blood sugar regulation. Potassium-rich foods, such as bitter melon and cinnamon, also have blood sugar-regulating properties. For instance, those who have trouble waking at night due to a blood sugar crash may actually benefit from 1 tablespoon of honey mixed with cinnamon before bed.

Vinegars are also shown to be supportive of regulating blood sugar when used prior to a meal.[9] Apple cider vinegar is most notably tolerated for this purpose, and having 1 tablespoon of raw apple cider vinegar before beginning a meal has been shown to drastically reduce blood glucose spikes.

While intermittent fasting and a ketogenic diet have been shown to drastically reduce and reverse insulin resistance, it's not recommended for cycling women with the goal of conception in mind, as carbohydrates are essential for the production of hormones.

In addition to dietary changes, lifestyle strategies can be supportive of healthy blood sugar, by changing the way the body tolerates glucose and insulin. For instance, movement after meals has been shown to regulate blood sugar. Regular sunlight exposure supports your circadian rhythm, which is essential for blood sugar management. Sunlight exposure also promotes healthy sleep patterns, which can negatively impact blood sugar when disrupted.

Stress is a major factor in the management of blood sugar and is not to be overlooked. Your diet may be perfect and your sleep on point, but if you are chronically stressed, you'll notice blood sugar handling is disrupted. For instance, you might notice that you experience a blood sugar spike in response to giving a presentation at work. This is your body's way of mobilizing glucose from a "paleolithic perspective," going back to the time of our ancient ancestors, where stress meant that we were in physical danger and likely needed to run away from something. Our bodies are incredibly intelligent but unable to differentiate between an emotional stress and a true threat, and as such will mobilize glucose to support us when needed.

Exercise is another strategy for blood sugar health, and it follows a "Goldilocks rule" where you're aiming for the perfect amount. Strength training and the building of muscle mass increase insulin sensitivity. However, too much exercise actually puts excess stress on the body that can negatively affect blood sugar the same way that other stressors can. Finding the perfect amount for you to support muscle mass, without depleting you, is important and will vary from person to person.

Chapter 17
Preconception Planning

As we approach the end of this book, you may be wondering, "Where do I start and how do I begin addressing these concerns?" While we have addressed the systems that are impacted as part of toxin exposure in prior chapters, and how to best support a return to health in those systems, I hope that this chapter may serve as a summary blueprint for supporting fertility by incorporating all of the pieces of the puzzle.

Preconception Timeline

In a perfect world, we all hope to conceive as soon as possible. In practice, I often say that "women with infertility want to conceive yesterday." While I can completely empathize with years of hoping, waiting, and disappointment, I hope that by now I have conveyed the importance of reducing toxicity and ultimately, detoxification of the things we face in our modern world. Doing so not only benefits the ability to conceive, but the health of your pregnancy as well as the health of your future child.

It's for that reason that patience is required when addressing these issues. In general, I recommend 6–12 months of preconception work before trying to conceive, with this work addressing the systems impacted by toxicity, as well as supporting appropriate detoxification. Some women get pregnant unexpectedly while reducing their toxicity, while others have greater detoxification needs and will need a longer period of time to clear their systems before they can begin trying to conceive.

Those who need a longer period of detoxification are often in the following situations:

- You have a history of digestive issues
- You have a history of thyroid abnormalities
- You have a diagnosis of insulin resistance, pre-diabetes, or diabetes
- You have a history of immune dysfunction
- Your menstrual cycle is irregular or absent
- You have a history of a diet lacking a core macronutrient (such as a vegan or carnivore diet)
- You have recently come off hormonal birth control
- You have recently had a child or are breastfeeding

If any of these apply to you, remember to be kind to yourself as you walk this journey and begin to support your body from a root cause approach. Your body has responded appropriately to its environment, and by reducing toxicity and supporting impacted systems, you'll be setting yourself up your success, whether you're hoping to conceive as soon as possible or years down the road.

Preconception Planning Checklist

The following are the most important factors to address when supporting fertility as it relates to your overall health. Each section has been broken down to assist you in determining if this area requires your support, and you can of course refer to the chapters dedicated to these topics throughout the book.

Opening drainage pathways

- Are you having a daily bowel movement that is a Type 3 of Type 4 on the Bristol Stool chart?
- Support liver drainage through food and lifestyle changes by incorporating coffee enemas, castor oil packs, and consuming healthy fats, as well as cruciferous vegetables and raw carrot salads.
- Consume half of your body weight in ounces of water daily plus the

addition of electrolytes, especially fulvic acid.

- Utilize dry brushing and get sweaty for skin detoxification.
- Incorporate breathing techniques to support lung detoxification and nervous system regulation.

Reducing toxicity

- Purchase organic, non-GMO produce when possible. If budget is a concern, focus on consuming the Clean 15 and avoiding the Dirty Dozen as outlined by the EWG each year to reduce pesticide consumption.
- Stop drinking tap water and switch to reverse osmosis at a minimum. For best results, and to remove all radioactive chemicals, invest in distilled water.
- Reduce the consumption of grains, including corn, rice, maize, and oats that frequently contain mycotoxins.
- Take air contamination in your home into account by investing in an air purification system that removes VOCs and mycotoxins from your indoor air. If this isn't in your budget, spend as much time outdoors as possible and routinely open the windows of your home to circulate fresh air, regardless of the season.
- Assess your kitchen and cookware to remove plastics, Teflon, and other harmful industrial chemicals involved in the cooking and storage of your food.
- Evaluate your personal care items including anything that goes in and on your body: menstrual care items, makeup, perfume, soap, shampoo, conditions, lotions, and facial care products. Consider replacing at least some of these items with alternatives that have fewer chemicals and toxins in them.
- Swap your conventional household cleaning products for natural products that don't introduce toxins into your home environment.
- Remember that everything does not need to happen at once. Replacing items as they run out is a good strategy for slowly incorporating healthy options as part of a non-toxic lifestyle.

Assessing and addressing mold

- If you suspect mold based on symptoms and your health history, order urine mycotoxin testing to screen for these poisonous substances. VCS testing can also be an affordable screening tool to rule out mycotoxin illness.
- If you suspect mold in your current home and have seen significant health changes since moving in, order an EMMA or ERMI to screen for dangerous mold and mycotoxins in your living environment. If found, find a professional remediation company to remove the issue.
- If you do have mycotoxins in urine testing, use the three-step approach to address it: support drainage, introduce binders, and utilize antifungals for colonization.

Address liver toxicity

- The liver is important for both gut and thyroid health, making it of utmost importance and one of the first impacted organ systems when the body is assaulted with toxicity.
- Assess for liver dysfunction based on symptoms, as well as blood chemistry testing, and support accordingly.

Restoring gut balance

- Support digestive capacity by utilizing hydrochloric acid, pancreatic enzymes, and bile support to ensure you are chemically digesting your food for maximum nutrient absorption.
- Assess the microbiome using comprehensive stool testing to determine beneficial bacterial status and pathogenic overgrowths in combination with presenting symptoms.
- Consider if eradication is necessary and what may be contributing to these overgrowths as well.

Revitalizing thyroid health

- Assess thyroid function via blood chemistry testing to screen for subclinical hypothyroidism, which can impact fertility.
- Nourish the thyroid with magnesium, zinc, selenium, and iodine.

- Consider toxins impacting the thyroid and reduce or eliminate them in your environment.
- If you also experience liver or gut dysfunction, address these, as they play an integral role in thyroid function.

Replenish nutrients

- Skip folic acid and supplement with methylfolate and other methylated B vitamins.
- Supplement 6–7 mg of magnesium per pound of body weight daily, spread throughout the day.
- Consume more omega-3 fatty acids in your diet or supplement with EPA and DHA ahead of conceiving, as well as throughout pregnancy.
- Supplement with 450 mg of choline daily if you have a history of miscarriage, as well as throughout pregnancy.
- Incorporate more vitamin A- and vitamin D-rich foods.
- Have your iron tested via blood chemistry and a full iron panel to determine if increased iron consumption is needed through diet or supplementation.
- Consider offsetting the impacts of glyphosate by consuming more glycine-rich foods in your diet.

Dietary strategies

- Focus on food quality over everything, but then consider balancing your meals to promote healthy blood sugar management.
- Consume plenty of cholesterol-rich foods to promote healthy sex hormone production.

Resources

Recommended Initial Blood Chemistry Testing

- CMP
- GGT
- CBC with differential
- Ferritin
- Total Iron
- TIBC
- % Iron Saturation
- Glucose
- Hemoglobin A1C
- Insulin
- LDH
- Vitamin D
- Magnesium RBC
- Uric Acid
- Homocysteine
- Lipid Panel
- Copper Serum
- Zinc Serum
- Ceruloplasmin

Resources for Additional Functional Testing

Vibrant America
www.vibrant-america.com

Mycotoxin urine testing
Heavy metal urine and blood testing
Industrial Chemicals and Pesticide urine testing

PFAS urine testing
Comprehensive blood chemistry testing
Gut Zoomer stool testing

Diagnostic Solutions
www.http://diagnosticsolutionslab.com

GI MAP stool testing

Mosaic (Formerly Great Plains Laboratory)
www.mosaicdx.com

MycoTOX urine testing
Glyphosate urine testing
Organic Acids Test (OAT) urine testing

Trace Elements
www.traceelements.com

Hair Tissue Mineral Analysis hair testing

Continuous Glucose Monitor

Direct access to a continuous glucose monitor (CGM) with an annual subscription and the ability to purchase sensors as you go, with the need for a diabetes diagnosis.

https://join.theiahealth.ai/c/always-growing

Acknowledgements

This book is a culmination of all the people who have loved and encouraged me unconditionally to make a difference in the lives of others. While my name is on the cover, these pages have been inspired by 10 years of hard work, continuing education, and clinical practice that have been possible thanks to the extraordinary, supportive people in my life.

Put simply, this book would not have been possible if it weren't for my human, my husband. Chris, you've been my biggest supporter all these years, and none of what I do would be possible without your constant pursuit of my happiness. You have believed in me from day one and have invested so much in my work, from putting your car up as collateral to fund my education to helping me take the time to write. For every person I am able to help, I hope they know that you are the driving force behind it.

Jasper, you have been the pinnacle of my life and most certainly of my career. Your eczema brought me to my lowest and most desperate point, and inspired me to shine a light on these topics for future mothers to help prevent their children from the same misery. You have taught me more in your short three years of life than I'll ever be able to teach you, and inadvertently, you have catapulted my career. Everything I do is for you.

I could not have done this without the support and expertise of my team, who has encouraged me every step of the way and is always pushing me to step out of my comfort zone to reach new heights. Anna McKelvey: your friendship and camaraderie have been a lighthouse for the past five years. Michelle Tierney: your brilliant mind was the force to be reckoned with behind this book, and your input made this it the masterpiece that it is. Julia Mims: I have learned so much from you as a mother and practitioner that went into these pages. Juliet Dalton: I am inspired by your love of deep research and wanted to translate that here. Elise Doppel: your organization and dedication to details helped me ensure nothing slipped through the cracks. Sara Mahan: the light within you inspired me to ensure that more than just the tangibles were discussed here. None of this would be possible without this team of women behind me as colleagues and friends.

Ashley Martucci: you're not only instrumental in our back-end administration, but you have seen me through the past 10 years as I dreamed of building a business, writing a book, and becoming a mother. You've seen it all, and your unwavering love has been a constant force in where we've ended up today.

Thank you to The Self Publishing Agency - Megan, Ira, and the whole team - for managing me within my hectic schedule to keep all the balls juggled in the air. A special thank you to my editor, Kathie Lynas, for diligently reviewing every detail to ensure we delivered the highest quality possible in this piece. This work would not be as refined as it is without your attention to detail and pushing me to ensure the content is digestible for all intended audiences.

Thank you to Restorative Wellness Solutions for providing me with the very best education for understanding the body comprehensively and building protocols that work. Your program is the reason I can confidently help anyone with any health issue.

Thank you to Dr. Jay and Dr. Todd from CellCore Biosciences. While your company looks like a supplement company to the outside world, I've wholeheartedly believe that it is actually an educational company and has drastically informed the way I practice.

References

Part One: The Root Cause of Fertility Challenges

Chapter 1: A Challenge for Our Times: Declining Fertility

1. Chandra, A., Copen, C.E., & Stephen, E.H. (2013). Infertility and Impaired Fecundity in the United States, 1982-2010: Data From the National Survey of Family Growth. *National Health Statistics Reports*, 67, 1-19. https://www.cdc.gov/nchs/data/nhsr/nhsr067.pdf (PDF 328 KB)
2. Leslie SW, Soon-Sutton TL, Khan MAB. Male Infertility. 2023 Mar 3. In: *StatPearls*. Treasure Island (FL): StatPearls Publishing; 2024 Jan–. PMID: 32965929.
3. Deshpande, P. S. & Gupta, A. S. (2019). Causes and Prevalence of Factors Causing Infertility in a Public Health Facility. *Journal of Human Reproductive Sciences*, 12(4): 287–293.
4. Swan, S. H. (2021). *Count Down: How Our Modern World Is Threatening Sperm Counts, Altering Male and Female Reproductive Development, and Imperiling the Future of the Human Race*. Scribner.
5. Strauss, J., Barbeiri, R. (2019). *Yen and Jaffe's Reproductive Endocrinology: Physiology, Pathology, and Clinical Management*. (6th ed.). Elsevier Inc.

Chapter 2: Surrounded by Unprecedented Toxicity

1. Environmental Working Group. (2005, July). The Body Burden: Pollution in Newborns. https://www.ewg.org/research/body-burden-pollution-newborns (Accessed September 10, 2023).
2. United States Environmental Protection Agency. (2024). *Toxic Substances Control Act Chemical Substance Inventory. Retrieved from https://www.epa.gov/tsca-inventory/*how-access-tsca-inventory.

3. Same as above.
4. Government Accountability Office: Chemical Regulation: Actions are Needed to Improve the Effectiveness of EPA's Chemical Review Program GAO-06-1032T: Published: Aug 2, 2006
5. National Institute of Health Sciences. (n.d.) Endocrine Disruptors. https://www.niehs.nih.gov/health/topics/agents/endocrine (Accessed September 9, 2023).
6. Colborn, T., Dumanoski, D., & Myers, J. P. (1997). *Our stolen future.* Abacus.
7. The Endocrine Disruptor Exchange. TEDX List of Potential Endocrine Disruptors. 2018. Available form http://www.endocrine-disruption.org/ (Accessed April 10, 2018).
8. Di Nisio, A., Polletta, L., Arisi, I., de Felice, B., & Falconi, M. (2018). Endocrine disruption of androgenic activity by perfluoroalkyl substances: Clinical and experimental evidence. *The Journal of Clinical Endocrinology & Metabolism*, 104(4), 1259-1271
9. Liew, Z., Luo, J., Nohr, E. A., Bech, B. H., Bossi, R., Arah, O. A., & Olsen, J. (2020). Maternal Plasma Perfluoroalkyl Substances and Miscarriage: A Nested Case–Control Study in the Danish National Birth Cohort. *Environmental Health Perspectives.* Volume 128, Issue 4. https://ehp.niehs.nih.gov/doi/full/10.1289/EHP6202
10. Bellinger, D. C. (2011). A strategy for comparing the contributions of environmental chemicals and other risk factors to neurodevelopment of children. *Environmental Health Perspectives,* 120(4), 501-507.
11. Grandjean, P., & Landrigan, P. J. (2014). Neurobehavioural effects of developmental toxicity. *The Lancet Neurology,* 13(3): 330–338.

Chapter 3: Industrial Chemicals & Plastics

1. United States Environmental Protection Agency. (2024). *Toxic Substances Control Act Chemical Substance Inventory.* Retrieved from https://www.epa.gov/tsca-inventory/how-access-tsca-inventory.

2. U. S. Government Accountability Office. (2006). Chemical Regulation: Actions are Needed to Improve the Effectiveness of EPA's Chemical Review Program GAO-06-1032T.
3. Same as above.
4. Norris, C. (2016, September 21). What is chromium-6 and how did it infiltrate America's drinking water? *PBS*. https://www.pbs.org/newshour/science/chromium-6-wash-many-drinking-supplies
5. Haelle, T. (2017, March 24). Asbestos still causes cancer. Why is it still used? *Forbes*. https://www.forbes.com/sites/tarahaelle/2017/03/24/asbestos-linked-cancer-remains-a-killer-just-as-asbestos-remains-commonly-used/#34691b033314
6. Petrlík, J., Behnisch, P., & DiGangi, J., et al. (2018) . Toxic Soup: Dioxins in Plastic Toys. *Arnika*. https://www.env-health.org/wp-content/uploads/2018/11/Toxic_Soup_brochure_en_web04-1.pdf
7. Guy, R. H. (2010). Predicting the rate and extent of fragrance chemical absorption into and through the skin. *Chemical research in toxicology*, 23(5), 864-870.
8. National Research Council. (2008). Phthalate Exposure Assessment in Humans.https://www.ncbi.nlm.nih.gov/books/NBK215044/ (Accessed August 17, 2023).
9. National Research Council. (2009). Phthalates and Cumulative Risk Assessment: The Tasks Ahead. *National Academies Press*. https://pubmed.ncbi.nlm.nih.gov/25009926/
10. Woodruff, T. J., Zota, A. R., & Schwartz, J. M. (2011). Environmental chemicals in pregnant women in the United States: NHANES 2003-2004. *Environmental Health Perspectives*, 119(6), 878.
11. Kumar, N., Srivastava, S., & Roy, P. (2015). Impact of low molecular weight phthalates in inducing reproductive malfunctions in male mice: Special emphasis on Sertoli cell functions. *General and Comparative Endocrinology*, 215, 36-50.
12. Latini, G., et al. (2006). Phthalate exposure and male infertility. *Toxicology*, 226(2-3), 90-98.

13. Kumar, N., et al. (2014). Assessment of estrogenic potential of diethyl phthalate in female reproductive system involving both genomic and non-genomic actions. *Reproductive Toxicology*, 49, 12-26.
14. Kay, V. R., Chambers, C., & Foster, W. G. (2013). Reproductive and developmental effects of phthalate diesters in females. *Critical Reviews in Toxicology*, 43(3), 200-219.
15. Trasande, L., et al. (2013). Urinary phthalates and increased insulin resistance in adolescents. *Pediatrics*, 132(3), e646-e655.
16. Boberg, J., et al. (2008). Impact of diisobutyl phthalate and other PPAR agonists on steroidogenesis and plasma insulin and leptin levels in fetal rats. *Toxicology*, 250(2), 75-81.
17. Stahlhut, R. W., et al. (2007). Concentrations of urinary phthalate metabolites are associated with increased waist circumference and insulin resistance in adult US males. *Environmental Health Perspectives*, 115, 876-882.
18. Parks, L. G., et al. (2000). The plasticizer diethylhexyl phthalate induces malformations by decreasing fetal testosterone synthesis during sexual differentiation in the male rat. *Toxicological Sciences*, 58(2), 339-349.
19. Lehmann, K. P., et al. (2004). Dose-dependent alterations in gene expression and testosterone synthesis in the fetal testes of male rats exposed to di (n-butyl) phthalate. *Toxicological Sciences*, 81(1), 60-68.
20. Faniband, M., Lindh, C. H., & Jönsson, B. A. G. (2014). Human biological monitoring of suspected endocrine-disrupting compounds. *Asian Journal of Andrology*, 16(1), 5.
21. Boberg, J., et al. (2010). Possible endocrine disrupting effects of parabens and their metabolites. *Reproductive Toxicology*, 30(2), 301-312.
22. Prusakiewicz, J. J., et al. (2007). Parabens inhibit human skin estrogen sulfotransferase activity: Possible link to paraben estrogenic effects. *Toxicology*, 232(3), 248-256.
23. Tavares, R. S., et al. (2009). Parabens in male infertility—Is there a mitochondrial connection? *Reproductive Toxicology*, 27(1), 1-7.

24. Byford, J. R., et al. (2002). Oestrogenic activity of parabens in MCF7 human breast cancer cells. *The Journal of Steroid Biochemistry and Molecular Biology,* 80(1), 49-60.
25. Wróbel, A. M., & Gregoraszczuk, E. Ł. (2014). Differential effect of methyl-, butyl-and propylparaben and 17β-estradiol on selected cell cycle and apoptosis gene and protein expression in MCF-7 breast cancer cells and MCF-10A non-malignant cells. *Journal of Applied Toxicology,* 34(9), 1041-1050.
26. Nishihama, Y., et al. (2016). Association between paraben exposure and menstrual cycle in female university students in Japan. *Reproductive Toxicology,* 63, 107-113.
27. Darbre, P. D., et al. (2004). Concentrations of parabens in human breast tumors. *Journal of Applied Toxicology,* 24(1), 5-13.
28. Calafat, A. M., et al. (2005). Urinary concentrations of bisphenol A and 4-nonylphenol in a human reference population. *Environmental Health Perspectives,* Advance online publication, 391-395.
29. Wilson, N. K., et al. (2007). An observational study of the potential exposures of preschool children to pentachlorophenol, bisphenol-A, and nonylphenol at home and daycare. *Environmental Research,* 103(1), 9-20.
30. Nadal, A., et al. (2009). The pancreatic β-cell as a target of estrogens and xenoestrogens: Implications for blood glucose homeostasis and diabetes. *Molecular and Cellular Endocrinology,* 304(1), 63-68.
31. Washam, C. (2006). Exploring the roots of diabetes: Bisphenol A may promote insulin resistance. *Environmental Health Perspectives,* 114(1), A48.
32. Boucher, J. G., et al. (2015). In Vitro Effects of Bisphenol A [beta]-D-Glucuronide (BPA-G) on Adipogenesis in Human and Murine Preadipocytes. *Environmental Health Perspectives,* 123(12), 1287.
33. Doherty, L. F., et al. (2010). In utero exposure to diethylstilbestrol (DES) or bisphenol-A (BPA) increases EZH2 expression in the mammary gland: An epigenetic mechanism linking endocrine disruptors to breast cancer. *Hormones and Cancer,* 1(3), 146-155.

34. Lathi, R. B., et al. (2014). Conjugated bisphenol A in maternal serum in relation to miscarriage risk. *Fertility and Sterility*, 102(1), 123-128.
35. Nah, W. H., Park, M. J., & Gye, M. C. (2011). Effects of early prepubertal exposure to bisphenol A on the onset of puberty, ovarian weights, and estrous cycle in female mice. *Clinical and Experimental Reproductive Medicine*, 38(2), 75-81.
36. Meeker, J. D., et al. (2010). Semen quality and sperm DNA damage in relation to urinary bisphenol A among men from an infertility clinic. *Reproductive Toxicology*, 30(4), 532-539.
37. Miao, M., et al. (2011). In utero exposure to bisphenol-A and its effect on birth weight of offspring. *Reproductive Toxicology*, 32(1), 64-68.
38. DeLuca, J. A. A., et al. (2018). Bisphenol-A alters microbiota metabolites derived from aromatic amino acids and worsens disease activity during colitis. *Experimental Biology and Medicine*, 243(10), 864-875.
39. Zalko, D., Jacques, C., Duplan, H., Bruel, S., & Perdu, E. (2011). Viable skin efficiently absorbs and metabolizes bisphenol A. *Chemosphere*, 82(3):424-30.
40. Qiu, W., et al. (2015). Actions of bisphenol A and bisphenol S on the reproductive neuroendocrine system during early development in zebrafish. *Endocrinology*, 157(2), 636-647.
41. Rochester, J. R., & Bolden, A. L. (2015). Bisphenol S and F: A systematic review and comparison of the hormonal activity of bisphenol A substitutes. *Environmental Health Perspectives*, 123(7), 643.
42. Chen, X., et al. (2014). Toxicity and estrogenic endocrine disrupting activity of phthalates and their mixtures. International *Journal of Environmental Research and Public Health*, 11(3), 3156-3168.
43. Sax, L. (2009). Polyethylene terephthalate may yield endocrine disruptors. *Environmental Health Perspectives*, 118(4), 445-448.

44. Wagner, M., & Oehlmann, J. (2011). Endocrine disruptors in bottled mineral water: Estrogenic activity in the E-Screen. The *Journal of Steroid Biochemistry and Molecular Biology,* 127(1-2), 128-135.
45. Greifenstein, M., et al. (2013). Impact of temperature and storage duration on the chemical and odor quality of military packaged water in polyethylene terephthalate bottles. *Science of the Total Environment,* 456, 376-383.
46. Aghaee, E. M., et al. (2014). Effects of storage time and temperature on the antimony and some trace element release from polyethylene terephthalate (PET) into the bottled drinking water. *Journal of Environmental Health Science and Engineering,* 12(1), 133.
47. Agency for Toxic Substances and Disease Registry. (2021, February). Antimony. https://wwwn.cdc.gov/TSP/substances/ToxSubstance.aspx?toxid=58 (Accessed September 11, 2023).
48. Loyo-Rosales, J. E., et al. (2004). Migration of nonylphenol from plastic containers to water and a milk surrogate. *Journal of Agricultural and Food Chemistry,* 52(7), 2016-2020.
49. Wagoner, J. K. (1983). Toxicity of vinyl chloride and poly (vinyl chloride): A critical review. *Environmental Health Perspectives,* 52, 61-66.
50. Calafat, A. M., et al. (2007). Polyfluoroalkyl chemicals in the US population: Data from the National Health and Nutrition Examination Survey (NHANES) 2003-2004 and comparisons with NHANES 1999-2000. *Environmental Health Perspectives,* 1596-1602.
51. Bossi, R., et al. (2005). Preliminary screening of perfluorooctane sulfonate (PFOS) and other fluorochemicals in fish, birds and marine mammals from Greenland and the Faroe Islands. *Environmental Pollution,* 136(2), 323-329.
52. Olsen, G. W., et al. (2007). Half-life of serum elimination of perfluorooctanesulfonate, perfluorohexanesulfonate, and perfluorooctanoate in retired fluorochemical production workers. *Environmental Health Perspectives,* 1298-1305.

53. Hunter, J. R., et al. (1992). Fecundity, spawning, and maturity of female Dover sole Microstomus pacificus, with an evaluation of assumptions and precision. *Fishery Bulletin*, 90(1), 101-128.
54. La Rocca, C., et al. (2012). Exposure and effective dose biomarkers for perfluorooctane sulfonic acid (PFOS) and perfluorooctanoic acid (PFOA) in infertile subjects: Preliminary results of the PREVIENI project. *International Journal of Hygiene and Environmental Health*, 215(2), 206-211.
55. Joensen, U. N., et al. (2009). Do perfluoroalkyl compounds impair human semen quality? *Environmental Health Perspectives*, 117(6), 923.
56. Cheng, Yan, et al. (2010) The Endocrine Disrupting Effect of Perfluorooctanoic Acid (PFOA) on Human Estrogen, Androgen and Thyroid Receptors. *Scientific Research*. Conference on Environmental Pollution and Public Health.
57. Knox, S. S., et al. (2011). Perfluorocarbon exposure, gender and thyroid function in the C8 Health Project. *The Journal of Toxicological Sciences*, 36(4), 403-410.
58. U.S. Environmental Protection Agency. (2005). Draft risk assessment of the potential human health effects associated with exposure to perfluorooctanoic acids and its salts.
59. Apelberg, B. J., et al. (2007). Cord serum concentrations of perfluorooctane sulfonate (PFOS) and perfluorooctanoate (PFOA) in relation to weight and size at birth. *Environmental Health Perspectives*, 1670-1676.
60. Fei, C., et al. (2007). Perfluorinated chemicals and fetal growth: A study within the Danish National Birth Cohort. *Environmental Health Perspectives*, 1677-1682.
61. Johnson, P. I., et al. (2014). The Navigation Guide--Evidence-Based Medicine Meets Environmental Health: Systematic Review of Human Evidence for PFOA Effects on Fetal Growth. *Environmental Health Perspectives* (Online), 122(10), 1028.
62. Nicole, Wendee. (2020). PFAS and Miscarriage in Humans: Expanding a Sparse Evidence Base. *Environ Health Perspective*, 128(10): 104002.

63. Liew, Z., Luo, J., Nohr, E. A., Bech, B. H., Bossi, R., Arah, O. A., & Olsen, J. (2020). Maternal Plasma Perfluoroalkyl Substances and Miscarriage: A Nested Case–Control Study in the Danish National Birth Cohort. *Environmental Health Perspectives.* 128, 4.
64. Norbäck, D., et al. (1995). Asthmatic symptoms and volatile organic compounds, formaldehyde, and carbon dioxide in dwellings. *Occupational and Environmental Medicine,* 52(6), 388-395.
65. Environmental Protection Agency. (2023). Volatile Organic Compounds' Impact on Indoor Air Quality. https://www.epa.gov/indoor-air-quality-iaq/volatile-organic-compounds-impact-indoor-air-quality. (Accessed September 11, 2023).
66. Bolla, K. I. (1991). Neuropsychological assessment for detecting adverse effects of volatile organic compounds on the central nervous system. *Environmental Health Perspectives,* 95, 93.
67. Cherry, N., et al. (2008). Occupation and male infertility: Glycol ethers and other exposures. *Occupational and Environmental Medicine,* 65(10), 708-714.
68. Sallmén, M., et al. (1998). Time to pregnancy among the wives of men exposed to organic solvents. *Occupational and Environmental Medicine,* 55(1), 24-30.
69. Kolstad, H. A., et al. (1999). Change in semen quality and sperm chromatin structure following occupational styrene exposure. *International Archives of Occupational and Environmental Health,* 72(3), 135-141.
70. Eldesouki, M. A., et al. (2013). Study of the Effect of Occupational Exposure to Volatile Organic Compounds (VOC's) on Male Reproductive Hormones. *World Journal of Medical Sciences,* 8(1), 6-12.
71. Cherry, N., et al. (2008). Occupation and male infertility: Glycol ethers and other exposures. *Occupational and Environmental Medicine,* 65(10), 708-714.
72. Ritz, B., & Wilhelm, M. (2008). Ambient air pollution and adverse birth outcomes: Methodologic issues in an emerging field. *Basic & Clinical Pharmacology & Toxicology,* 102(2), 182-190.

73. Forand, S. P., Lewis-Michl, E. L., & Gomez, M. I. (2012). Adverse birth outcomes and maternal exposure to trichloroethylene and tetrachloroethylene through soil vapor intrusion in New York State. *Environmental Health Perspectives,* 120(4), 616.
74. Windham, G. C., et al. (2006). Autism spectrum disorders in relation to distribution of hazardous air pollutants in the San Francisco Bay area. *Environmental Health Perspectives,* 1438-1444.
75. Kalkbrenner, A. E., et al. (2010). Perinatal exposure to hazardous air pollutants and autism spectrum disorders at age 8. *Epidemiology* (Cambridge, Mass.), 21(5), 631.
76. Croen, L. A., et al. (1997). Maternal residential proximity to hazardous waste sites and risk for selected congenital malformations. *Epidemiology,* 8(4), 347-354.
77. McDonald, B. C., et al. (2018). Volatile chemical products emerging as largest petrochemical source of urban organic emissions. *Science,* 359(6377), 760-764.
78. Agency for Toxic Substances and Disease Registry (1998). Public Health Statement for 2- Butoxyethanol and 2-Butoxyethanol Acetate. https://www.atsdr.cdc.gov/ToxProfiles/tp118-c1-b.pdf. (Accessed September 11, 2023).
79. Same as above.
80. World Health Organization. (2016, March). Dioxins and Their Effects on Human Health. https://epawebapp.epa.ie/licences/lic_eDMS/090151b28007b07c.pdf. (Accessed September 10, 2023).
81. Birnbaum, L. S., & Fenton, S. E. (2003). Cancer and developmental exposure to endocrine disruptors. *Environmental Health Perspectives,* 111(4), 389.
82. Kohn, M. C., et al. (1996). A mechanistic model of effects of dioxin on thyroid hormones in the rat. *Toxicology and Applied Pharmacology,* 136(1), 29-48.
83. Same as above.
84. Birnbaum, L. S., & Fenton, S. E. (2003). Cancer and developmental exposure to endocrine disruptors. *Environmental Health Perspectives,* 111(4), 389.

85. Chen, Y.-J., et al. (2012). Progesterone receptor is involved in 2,3,7,8-tetrachlorodibenzo-p-dioxin-stimulated breast cancer cells proliferation. *Cancer Letters,* 319(2), 223-231.
86. Garry, V. F., et al. (2002). Birth defects, season of conception, and sex of children born to pesticide applicators living in the Red River Valley of Minnesota, USA. *Environmental Health Perspectives,* 110(Suppl 3), 441.
87. Neuberger, M., Schut, P., Himmelreich, A., Kundi, M., & Wallner, P. (1999). Persistent health effects of dioxin contamination in herbicide production. *Environmental Research,* 81(3), 206-214.
88. Kerkvliet, N. (1995). Immunological effects of chlorinated dibenzo-p-dioxins. *Environ Health Perspective.* 9 (9):47-53.
89. National Institute of Environmental Health Sciences. (2016, March). *Toxic Chemicals and Environmental Health Risk Where you Live and Work.*

Chapter 4: Heavy Metals

1. Sasaki, N. & Carpenter, D. (2022). Associations between Metal Exposures and Cognitive Function in American Older Adults. *International Journal of Environmental Research and Public Health.* 19(4): 2327.
2. Bakulski, K., et al. (2020). Heavy Metals Exposure and Alzheimer's Disease and Related Dementias. *Journal of Alzheimer Disease.* 76(4): 1215–1242.
3. National Organization for Rare Diseases. (2008). Heavy Metal Poisoning. https://rarediseases.org/rare-diseases/heavy-metal-poisoning/ (Accessed September 10, 2023).
4. Same as above.
5. Koszewicz, M., et al. (2021). The impact of chronic co-exposure to different heavy metals on small fibers of peripheral nerves. A study of metal industry workers. *Journal of Occupational Medicine and Toxicology.* 16: 12.
6. Smyth D, Kramarz C, Carr AS, et al. (2023). Toxic neuropathies: a practical approach. *Practical Neurology.* 23:120-130.

7. Pamphlett, R., et al. (2023). Potentially toxic elements in the brains of people with multiple sclerosis. *Scientific Reports.* 13: 655.
8. Gaioli, G., et al. (2020). Heavy metals in the enviroment: Guillain-Barre like syndrome. *Arch Argent Pediatr.*
9. Pyatha, S., et al. (2022). Association between Heavy Metal Exposure and Parkinson's Disease: A Review of the Mechanisms Related to Oxidative Stress. *Antioxidants.* 11(12): 2467.
10. Castellanos, M. & Fuente, A. (2016). The Adverse Effects of Heavy Metals with and without Noise Exposure on the Human Peripheral and Central Auditory System: A Literature Review. International *Journal of Environmental Research and Public Health.* 13(12): 1223.
11. Jaishankar, M., et al. (2014). Toxicity, mechanism and health effects of some heavy metals. *Interdisciplinary Toxicology.* 7(2): 60–72.
12. Austin, D.W., et al. (2014). Genetic Variation Associated with Hypersensitivity to Mercury. *Toxicology International.* 21(3): 236–241.
13. Ledda, C, et al. (2020). Exposure to Toxic Heavy Metals Can Influence Homocysteine Metabolism? *Antioxidants.* 9(1): 30.
14. D'Souza, H.S., et al. (2003). Role of essential trace minerals on the absorption of heavy metals with special reference to lead. Indian Journal of Clinical Biochemistry. 18(2): 154–160.
15. Giles, B. & Mann, K. (2022). Arsenic as an immunotoxicant. *Toxicology and Applied Pharmacology.* 454:116248.
16. Yang, Y., et al. (2023). Chronic Arsenic Exposure Perturbs Gut Microbiota and Bile Acid Homeostasis in Mice. *American Chemical Society.* 36, 7, 1037–1043
17. Tibau, A. V. & Grube, B. (2019). Mercury Contamination from Dental Amalgam. *Journal of Health and Pollution.* 9(22): 190612.
18. Aschner, M. & Aschner, J. L. (1990). Mercury neurotoxicity: mechanisms of blood-brain barrier transport. *Neuroscience and Behavioral Reviews.* 14(2):169-76.
19. Agency for Toxic Substances and Disease Control. (2023). *Lead toxicity.* https://www.atsdr.cdc.gov/csem/leadtoxicity/physiological_effects.

20. Rastogi, S.K. (2008). Renal effects of environmental and occupational lead exposure. *Indian Journal of Occupational and Environmental Medicine.* 12(3): 103–106.
21. Gundacker, C. & Hengstschläger, M. (2012). The role of the placenta in fetal exposure to heavy metals. *Wien Med Wochenschr.* 162, 201–206.
22. Wang, Q., et al. (2023). High dietary copper intake induces perturbations in the gut microbiota and affects host ovarian follicle development. *Ecotoxicology and Environmental Safety.* 255, 114810.
23. Darbre, P. D. (2006). Metalloestrogens: an emerging class of inorganic xenoestrogens with potential to add to the oestrogenic burden of the human breast. *Journal of Applied Toxicology.* 3:191-7.
24. Mehta, S.W. & Eikum, R. (1989). Effect of estrogen on serum and tissue levels of copper and zinc. *Advances in Experimental Medicine and Biology.* 258:155-62.
25. Beshir, S., et al. (2016). Hormonal Perturbations in Occupationally Exposed Nickel Workers. *Open Access Macedonian Journal of Medical Sciences.* 4(2): 307–311.
26. Darbre, P. D. (2005). Aluminium, antiperspirants and breast cancer. *Journal of Inorganic Biochemistry,* 99(9), 1912-1919.
27. Exley, C., Darbre, P. D., & Long, G. S. (2007). Aluminium in human breast tissue. *Journal of Inorganic Biochemistry,* 101(9), 1344-1346.
28. Darbre, P. D. (2006). Metalloestrogens: an emerging class of inorganic xenoestrogens with potential to add to the oestrogenic burden of the human breast. *Journal of Applied Toxicology,* 26(3), 191-197.
29. Romanowicz-Makowska, H., Forma, E., Bryś, M., Krajewska, W. M., Smolarz, B., & Krześlak, A. (2011). Concentration of cadmium, nickel and aluminium in female breast cancer. *Polish Journal of Pathology: Official Journal of the Polish Society of Pathologists,* 62(4), 257-261.
30. Sun, Q., et al. (2022). Heavy metals induced mitochondrial dysfunction in animals: Molecular mechanism of toxicity. *Toxicology.* 469:153136.

31. Yıldırım, E., & Derici, M. K. (2019). The Effect of Heavy Metals on Miscarriage. *Journal of Clinical Obstetrics and Gynecology*, 29(1), 31-38.
32. Omeljaniuk, W. J., et al. (2018). Cadmium and Lead in Women Who Miscarried. *Clinical Laboratory*, 64(1):59-67.
33. Kumar, V., & Gill, K. D. (2014). Oxidative stress and mitochondrial dysfunction in aluminium neurotoxicity and its amelioration: A review. *Neurotoxicology*, 41, 154-166.
34. Kumar, V., & Gill, K. D. (2009). Aluminium neurotoxicity: Neurobehavioural and oxidative aspects. *Archives of Toxicology*, 83(11), 965-978.
35. Anka, A., et al. (2022). Potential mechanisms of some selected heavy metals in the induction of inflammation and autoimmunity. *European Journal of Inflammation*. 20.
36. Witkowska, D., et al. (2021). Heavy Metals and Human Health: Possible Exposure Pathways and the Competition for Protein Binding Sites. *Molecules*, 26(19): 6060.
37. Aquino, N., et al. (2012). Role of Cadmium and Nickel in Estrogen Receptor Signaling and Breast Cancer: Metalloestrogens or Not? *Journal of Environmental Science and Health, Part C: Environmental Carcinogenesis and Ecotoxicology Reviews* 30(3): 189–224.
38. Liu, D., et al. (2023). Effects of Endocrine-Disrupting Heavy Metals on Human Health. *Toxics*. 11(4): 322.

Chapter 5: Radioactive Substances

1. Nobel, J. (2020). America's Radioactive Secret. Rolling Stone. Retried from https://www.rollingstone.com/politics/politics-features/oil-gas-fracking-radioactive-investigation-937389/
2. Hendrix, Glen. (2020). The Fracking Industry Is Selling Radioactive Waste Brine to the Public as a Road Deicer and Pool Treatment. *Medium*. Retrieved from https://medium.com/age-of-awareness/the-fracking-industry-is-selling-radioactive-waste-brine-to-the-public-as-a-road-deicer-and-pool-ba77a0f67e1d

3. Abramenkovs, A., et al. (2022). Ra-223 induces clustered DNA damage and inhibits cell survival in several prostate cancer cell lines. *Translation Oncology*, 26:101543.
4. Wang, S., et al. (2019). Review of Uranium-Induced Reproductive Toxicity. *Biological Trace Element Research*, 196, 204-213.
5. Agency for Toxic Substances and Disease Registry. (2014). Public Health Statement for Radium. *Center for Disease Control and Prevention*. Retrieved from https://wwwn.cdc.gov/TSP/PHS/PHS.aspx?phsid=789&toxid=154#:~:text=If%20radium%20is%20swallowed%20in,urine%20on%20a%20daily%20basis.
6. United States Geological Survey. (1998). Radium-226 and Radium-228 in Shallow Ground Water, Southern New Jersey. Retrieved from https://pubs.usgs.gov/fs/1998/0062/report.pdf
7. United States Environmental Protection Agency. (2023, August). Health Effects of Uranium. https://www.epa.gov/navajo-nation-uranium-cleanup/health-effects-uranium (Accessed September 9, 2023).
8. Grison, S., et al. (2022). Multigenerational Exposure to Uranium Changes Sperm Metabolome in Rats. *International Journal of Molecular Sciences*. 23(15): 8349.
9. Environmental Working Group.(2018(. EWG Interactive Radium Map. Retrieved from https://www.ewg.org/interactive-maps/2018-radium/
10. Environmental Working Group. (2018). *170 Million in U.S. Drink Radioactive Tap Water*. https://www.ewg.org/research/170-million-us-drink-radioactive-tap-water (Accessed September 9, 2023).
11. Same as above.
12. Agency for Toxic Substances and Disease Registry. (2014). Public Health Statement for Radium. *Center for Disease Control and Prevention*. Retrieved from https://wwwn.cdc.gov/TSP/PHS/PHS.aspx?phsid=789&toxid=154#:~:text=If%20radium%20is%20swallowed%20in,urine%20on%20a%20daily%20basis.
13. Ubios, A. M., et al. (1997). Skin alterations induced by long-term exposure to uranium and their effect on permeability. *Health Physics*, 72(5):713-5.

14. Song, S. & Lambert, P. (1999). Different Responses of Epidermal and Hair Follicular Cells to Radiation Correlate with Distinct Patterns of p53 and p21 Induction. *The American Journal of Pathology*, 155(4): 1121–1127.
15. Kim, S. E., et al. (2020). Effects of radiation therapy on the meibomian glands and dry eye in patients with ocular adnexal mucosa-associated lymphoid tissue lymphoma. *BMC Ophthalmology*, 20, 24.
16. Chalifoux, R. & Elisevich, K. (1996). Effect of ionizing radiation on partial seizures attributable to malignant cerebral tumors. *Stereotactic and Functional Neurosurgery*, 67(3-4):169-82.
17. Lie, L., et al. (2021). Bioaccumulation of uranium by Candida utilis: Investigated by water chemistry and biological effects. *Environmental Research*, 194:110691.
18. Domingo, J. L. (2001). Reproductive and developmental toxicity of natural and depleted uranium: a review. *Reproductive Toxicology*, 15(6):603-9.
19. Wang, S., et al. (2020). A Review of Uranium-Induced Reproductive Toxicity. *Biological Trace Element Research*, 196(1):204-213.
20. Environmental Protection Agency. (2014). "Uranium and Radiation on the Navajo Nation." Retrieved from https://www.epa.gov/sites/default/files/2016-06/documents/atsdr_uranium_and_radiation_health_dec_2014.pdf
21. Yang, Y., et al. (2024). Role of uranium toxicity and uranium-induced oxidative stress in advancing kidney injury and endothelial inflammation in rats. *BMC Pharmacology and Toxicology*, 25, 14.

Chapter 6: Pesticides & Herbicides

1. Dalvie, M., et al. (2004). The long-term effects of DDT exposure on semen, fertility, and sexual function of malaria vector-control workers in Limpopo Province, South Africa. *Environmental Research*. 96(1):1-8.

2. Herrero-Mercado, M., Waliszewski, S. M., Caba, M., & Martínez-Valenzuela, C. (2010). Organochlorine pesticide levels in umbilical cord blood of newborns in Veracruz, Mexico. *Bulletin of Environmental Contamination and Toxicology*, 85(4), 367-371.
3. Ouyang, F., et al. (2005). Serum DDT, age at menarche, and abnormal menstrual cycle length. *Occupational and Environmental Medicine*, 62(12), 878-884.
4. Cohn, B. A., Wolff, M. S., Cirillo, P. M., & Sholtz, R. I. (2003). DDT and DDE exposure in mothers and time to pregnancy in daughters. *The Lancet*, 361(9376), 2205-2206.
5. Younglai, E. V., Holloway, A. C., Foster, W. G., & Jarrell, J. F. (2002). Levels of environmental contaminants in human follicular fluid, serum, and seminal plasma of couples undergoing in vitro fertilization. *Archives of Environmental Contamination and Toxicology*, 43(1), 121-126.
6. Longnecker, M. P., Klebanoff, M. A., Brock, J. W., & Zhou, H. (2001). Association between maternal serum concentration of the DDT metabolite DDE and preterm and small-for-gestational-age babies at birth. *The Lancet*, 358(9276), 110-114.
7. Sagiv, S. K., Thurston, S. W., Bellinger, D. C., Tolbert, P. E., Altshul, L. M., Korrick, S. A. (2008). Prenatal organochlorine exposure and measures of behavior in infancy using the Neonatal Behavioral Assessment Scale (NBAS). *Environmental Health Perspectives*, 116(5), 666-673.
8. Al-Othman, A. A., Abd-Alrahman, S. H., & Al-Daghri, N. M. (2015). DDT and its metabolites are linked to increased risk of type 2 diabetes among Saudi adults: A cross-sectional study. *Environmental Science and Pollution Research*, 22(1), 379-386.
9. Brown, A. S., Cheslack-Postava, K., Rantakokko, P., Kiviranta, H., Hinkka-Yli-Salomäki, S., McKeague, I. W., ... & Sourander, A. (2018). Association of maternal insecticide levels with autism in offspring from a national birth cohort. *American Journal of Psychiatry*, 175(11), 1094-1101.

10. Agency for Toxic Substances and Disease Registry. (2022). ToxGuide for DDT, DDE, DDD. Retrieved from https://www.atsdr.cdc.gov/toxguides/toxguide-35.pdf
11. https://www.ncbi.nlm.nih.gov/pmc/articles/PMC5044953/
12. Environmental Working Group. (2023). *Glyphosate.* https://www.epa.gov/ingredients-used-pesticide-products/glyphosate. (Accessed September 8 , 2023).
13. Same as above.
14. Mills, P. J., Kania-Korwel, I., Fagan, J., McEvoy, L. K., Laughlin, G. A., Barrett-Connor, E., ... & Nowakowski, S. (2017). Excretion of the herbicide glyphosate in older adults between 1993 and 2016. *JAMA,* 318(16), 1610-1611.
15. Savitz, D. A., et al. (1997). Male pesticide exposure and pregnancy outcome. *American Journal of Epidemiology,* 146(12), 1025-1036.
16. Cattani, D., et al. (2014). Mechanisms underlying the neurotoxicity induced by glyphosate-based herbicide in immature rat hippocampus: involvement of glutamate excitotoxicity. *Toxicology,* 320, 34-45.
17. Thongprakaisang, S., et al. (2013). Glyphosate induces human breast cancer cells growth via estrogen receptors. *Food and Chemical Toxicology,* 59, 129-136.
18. Garry, V. F., et al. (2002). Birth defects, season of conception, and sex of children born to pesticide applicators living in the Red River Valley of Minnesota, USA. *Environmental Health Perspectives,* 110(Suppl 3), 441.
19. Kurenbach, B., et al. (2015). Sublethal exposure to commercial formulations of the herbicides dicamba, 2,4-dichlorophenoxyacetic acid, and glyphosate cause changes in antibiotic susceptibility in Escherichia coli and Salmonella enterica serovar Typhimurium. mBio, 6(2), e00009-15.
20. Center for Disease Control, (2024). *2019 Antibiotic Resistance Threats Report.* Retrieved from https://www.cdc.gov/antimicrobial-resistance/data-research/threats/index.html

21. Jacob, G.S., et al. (1988). Metabolism of glyphosate in Pseudomonas sp. strain LBr. *Applied and Environmental Microbiology*. 54(12): 2953–2958.
22. Larsen, K., et al. (2012). Effects of sub-lethal exposure of rats to the herbicide glyphosate in drinking water: Glutathione transferase enzyme activities, levels of reduced glutathione and lipid peroxidation in liver, kidneys and small intestine. *Environmental Toxicology and Pharmacology*, 34(3), 811-818.
23. Fath, M.A., et al. (2020). Disruption of cytochrome P450 enzymes in the liver and small intestine in chicken embryos in ovo exposed to glyphosate. *Environmental Science and Pollution Research*. 27(14):16865-16875.
24. Park, Y., et al. (2014). The Simplest Flowchart Stating the Mechanisms for Organic Xenobiotics-induced Toxicity: Can it Possibly be Accepted as a "Central Dogma" for Toxic Mechanisms? *Toxicological Research*. 30(3): 179–184.
25. El-Shenawy, N. S. (2009). Oxidative stress responses of rats exposed to Roundup and its active ingredient glyphosate. *Environmental Toxicology and Pharmacology*, 28(3):379-85.
26. Mills, P., et al. (2019). Glyphosate Excretion is Associated With Steatohepatitis and Advanced Liver Fibrosis in Patients With Fatty Liver Disease. *Clinical Gastroenterology and Hepatology*. 3: 741-743.
27. Peillex, C. & Pelletier, M. (2020). The impact and toxicity of glyphosate and glyphosate-based herbicides on health and immunity. *Journal of Immunotoxicology*. 17(1):163-174.
28. Same as above.
29. Winstone, J., et al. (2022). Glyphosate infiltrates the brain and increases pro-inflammatory cytokine TNFα: implications for neurodegenerative disorders. *Journal of Neuroinflammation*. 19(1):193.
30. Vojdani, A., et al. (2020). Interaction between food antigens and the immune system: Association with autoimmune disorders. *Autoimmunity Reviews*. 19(3).

31. Munos, J., et al. (2021). Glyphosate and the key characteristics of an endocrine disruptor: A review. *Chemosphere*. 270.
32. Serra, L., et al. (2021). Review: Mechanisms of Glyphosate and Glyphosate-Based Herbicides Action in Female and Male Fertility in Humans and Animal Models. *Cells*. 10(11), 3079.
33. Beecham, J. E., & Seneff, S. (2016). Is there a link between autism and glyphosate-formulated herbicides? *Journal of Autism*, 3(1), 1.
34. Kwong, T. C. (2002). Organophosphate pesticides: Biochemistry and clinical toxicology. *Therapeutic Drug Monitoring*, 24(1), 144-149.
35. Behan, P. O. (1996). Chronic fatigue syndrome as a delayed reaction to chronic low-dose organophosphate exposure. *Journal of Nutritional & Environmental Medicine*, 6(4), 341-350.
36. Bouchard, M. F., et al. (2011). Prenatal exposure to organophosphate pesticides and IQ in 7-year-old children. *Environmental Health Perspectives*, 119(8), 1189.
37. Eskenazi, B., Bradman, A., & Castorina, R. (1999). Exposures of children to organophosphate pesticides and their potential adverse health effects. *Environmental Health Perspectives*, 107(Suppl 3), 409.
38. Bouchard, M. F., et al. (2010). Attention-deficit/hyperactivity disorder and urinary metabolites of organophosphate pesticides. *Pediatrics*, 125(6), e1270-e1277.
39. Meeker, J. D., et al. (2006). Exposure to nonpersistent insecticides and male reproductive hormones. *Epidemiology*, 17(1), 61-68.
40. Recio, R., et al. (2005). Pesticide exposure alters follicle-stimulating hormone levels in Mexican agricultural workers. *Environmental Health Perspectives*, 113, 1160-1163.
41. Pesticide National Synthesis Project. (2024). https://water.usgs.gov/nawqa/pnsp/usage/maps/compound_listing.php?year=2016&hilo=L. (Accessed March 1, 2024).
42. Joly, C., et al. (2013). Impact of chronic exposure to low doses of chlorpyrifos on the intestinal microbiota in the Simulator of the Human Intestinal Microbial Ecosystem (SHIME®) and in the rat. *Environmental Science and Pollution Research*, 20(5), 2726-2734.

43. Zhao, Y., et al. (2016). Effects of chlorpyrifos on the gut microbiome and urine metabolome in mouse (Mus musculus). *Chemosphere,* 153, 287-293.
44. Gore, A. (2002). Organochlorine pesticides directly regulate gonadotropin-releasing hormone gene expression and biosynthesis in the GT1-7 hypothalamic cell line. *Molecular and Cellular Endocrinology.* 192(1-2):157-70.
45. Foradori, C., et al. (2011). The Differential Effect of Atrazine on Luteinizing Hormone Release in Adrenalectomized Adult Female Wistar Rats. *Biology of Reproduction.* 85 (4), 684–689.
46. Wirbisky, S. & Freeman, J. (2015). Atrazine Exposure and Reproductive Dysfunction through the Hypothalamus-Pituitary-Gonadal (HPG) Axis. *Toxics.* 3(4), 414-450.
47. Hayes, T., et al. (2010). Atrazine induces complete feminization and chemical castration in male African clawed frogs (Xenopus laevis). *Proceedings of the National Academy of Sciences.* 107(10): 4612–4617.

Chapter 7: Mold & Mycotoxins

1. Ballo, A., et al. (2023). Estrogenic and Non-Estrogenic Disruptor Effect of Zearalenone on Male Reproduction: A Review. *International Journal of Molecular Sciences,* 24(2), 1578.
2. Mostrom, M. (2021). Mycotoxin-Associated Estrogenism and Vulvovaginitis in Animals. Merck Manual Veterinary Manual. Retrieved from https://www.merckvetmanual.com/toxicology/mycotoxicoses/mycotoxin-associated-estrogenism-and-vulvovaginitis-in-animals#
3. Jafari-Nodoushan, A. A. (2022). Zearalenone, an abandoned mycoestrogen toxin, and its possible role in human infertility. *International Journal of Reproductive Biomedicine,* 20(2): 151–153.
4. Yip, K. Y., et al. (2017). Combined low-dose zearalenone and aflatoxin B1 on cell growth and cell-cycle progression in breast cancer MCF-7 cells. *Toxicology Letters,* 281:139-151.

5. Li, R., et al. (2020). Dietary exposure to mycotoxin zearalenone (ZEA) during post-implantation adversely affects placental development in mice. *Reproductive Toxicology*, 85: 42–50.
6. Water Mold Fire Restoration. (n.d.). *Twelve Important Mold Statistics for 2021*. Retrieved from https://watermoldfire.net/important-mold-statistics/
7. Klinghardt, D. (2000). Metal Toxicity. Retrieved from https://klinghardtinstitute.com/wp-content/uploads/2023/05/Metal-Toxicity.pdf
8. Pierron, A., et al. (2016). Impact of mycotoxin on immune response and consequences for pig health. *Animal Nutrition*, 2(2): 63–68.
9. Jeffery, F. H., et al. (1984). Effects of some clinically significant mycotoxins on the incorporation of DNA, RNA and protein precursors in cultured mammalian cells. *Research in Veterinary Science*, 37(1):30-8.
10. Guilford, T. & Hope, J. (2014). Deficient Glutathione in the Pathophysiology of Mycotoxin-Related Illness. *Toxins*, 6(2): 608–623.
11. Gonkowski, S., et al. (2020). Mycotoxins and the Enteric Nervous System. *Toxins*. 12(7): 461.
12. Jedrychowski, W., et al. (2011). Cognitive function of 6-year old children exposed to mold-contaminated homes in early postnatal period. Prospective birth cohort study in Poland. *Physiology & Behavior*. 104(5):989-95.
13. Ratnaseelan, A., et al. (2018). Effects of Mycotoxins on Neuropsychiatric Symptoms and Immune Processes. *Clinical Therapeutics*, 40(6):903-917.

Part Two: Restoring Whole Body Health to Support Fertility

Chapter 8: Clearing Your Body of Toxins: The Critical Role of Drainage

1. Peterson, C. T., et al. (2017). Therapeutic Uses of Triphala in Ayurvedic Medicine. *Journal of Alternative and Complementary Medicine*. 23(8): 607–614.
2. Nariya, M., et al. (2009). Comparison of enteroprotective efficacy of triphala formulations (Indian Herbal Drug) on methotrexate-induced small intestinal damage in rats. *Phytotherapy Research*. 23(8):1092-8.
3. Hundt, M., et al. (2022). Physiology, Bile Secretion. *StatPearls*, Treasure Island (FL): StatPearls Publishing.
4. Gupta, V. K., & Aggarwal, B. B. (2014). Therapeutic potential of castor oil and its active constituent ricinoleic acid. *Expert Opinion on Investigational Drugs*, 23(1), 11-30.
5. Same as above.
6. Kreitzer, M. J., & Gross, A. E. (2008). Castor oil packs for the treatment of chronic constipation: A pilot study. *Integrative Cancer Therapies*, 7(4), 327-332.
7. Magner, L. (1992). *A History of Medicine*. Boca Raton, Florida: CRC Press.
8. Friedenwald, J., & Morrison, S. (1940, February). The history of the enema with some notes on related procedures (Part II). *Bulletin of the History of Medicine*, 8(2), 239–276.
9. Museum of Quackery. "Dr. John Harvey Kellogg." *Great American Quacks*. Retrieved 12 February 2023.
10. The Gerson Institute. (2003). "Alternative Cancer Treatment." Gerson Therapy. Retrieved from https://web.archive.org/web/20030401121651/http://gerson.org/g_therapy/default.asp

11. Mehta, S. (2018). A study to assess the effectiveness of rebounding exercise on lymphedema. *Indian Journal of Physical Therapy and Rehabilitation.*
12. Sears, M. E., Kerr, K. J., & Bray, R. I. (2012). Arsenic, cadmium, lead, and mercury in sweat: A systematic review. *Journal of Environmental and Public Health,* 2012.
13. Hohnadel, D. C., et al. (1973). Atomic absorption spectrometry of nickel, copper, zinc, and lead in sweat collected from healthy subjects during sauna bathing. *Clinical Chemistry,* 19(11), 1288-1292.
14. Genuis, S. J., et al. (2011). Blood, urine, and sweat (BUS) study: Monitoring and elimination of bioaccumulated toxic elements. *Archives of Environmental Contamination and Toxicology,* 61(2), 344-357.
15. Genuis, S. J., Lane, K., & Birkholz, D. (2016). Human elimination of organochlorine pesticides: Blood, urine, and sweat study. *BioMed Research International,* 2016.
16. Patrick, R. & Johnson, T. (2021). Sauna use as a lifestyle practice to extend healthspan. *Experimental Gerontology.* 154(15).
17. Webster, E. (2022). The Impact of Adverse Childhood Experiences on Health and Development in Young Children. *Global Pediatric Health.* 9.
18. Zhang, Z. (2022). Om chanting modulates the processing of negative stimuli: Behavioral and electrophysiological evidence. *Frontiers in Psychology,* 13.
19. Bach, D., et al. (2019). Clinical EFT (Emotional Freedom Techniques) Improves Multiple Physiological Markers of Health. *Journal of Evidence-Based Integrative Medicine.* 24.
20. Davey, S., et al. (2021). Where is emotional feeling felt in the body? An integrative review. *PLOS.*

Chapter 9: Reducing Exposure Sources

1. Schecter, A., et al. (2008). Brominated flame retardants in US food. *Molecular Nutrition & Food Research,* 52(2), 266-272.

2. The Endogenous Hormones and Breast Cancer Collaborative Group. (2010). Insulin-like growth factor 1 (IGF1), IGF binding protein 3 (IGFBP3), and breast cancer risk: pooled individual data analysis of 17 prospective studies. *The Lancet Oncology*, 11(6), 530-542.
3. Peyrat, J. P., et al. (1993). Plasma insulin-like growth factor-1 (IGF-1) concentrations in human breast cancer. *European Journal of Cancer*, 29(4), 492-497.
4. Mantzoros, C. S., et al. (1997). Insulin-like growth factor 1 in relation to prostate cancer and benign prostatic hyperplasia. *British Journal of Cancer*, 76(9), 1115.
5. Probst-Hensch, N. M., et al. (2001). IGF-1, IGF-2 and IGFBP-3 in prediagnostic serum: association with colorectal cancer in a cohort of Chinese men in Shanghai. *British Journal of Cancer*, 85(11), 1695.
6. Van Elswyk, M. E., & McNeill, S. H. (2014). Impact of grass/forage feeding versus grain finishing on beef nutrients and sensory quality: The US experience. *Meat Science*, 96(1), 535-540.
7. McAfee, A. J., et al. (2011). Red meat from animals offered a grass diet increases plasma and platelet n-3 PUFA in healthy consumers. *British Journal of Nutrition*, 105(1), 80-89.
8. Daley, C. A., et al. (2010). A review of fatty acid profiles and antioxidant content in grass-fed and grain-fed beef. *Nutrition Journal*, 9(1), 10.
9. The Organic Center. (n.d.). The Benefits of Organic Meat. The Organic Network. Retrieved from https://www.organic-center.org/no-synthetic-growth-promoters-organic-meat
10. Coletta, J. M., Bell, S. J., & Roman, A. S. (2010). Omega-3 fatty acids and pregnancy. *Reviews in Obstetrics and Gynecology*, 3(4), 163.
11. Oster, E. (2013). *Expecting Better: Why the Conventional Pregnancy Wisdom is Wrong - and What You Really Need to Know*. New York, NY: Penguin Books.
12. Hibbeln, J. R., et al. (2007). Maternal seafood consumption in pregnancy and neurodevelopmental outcomes in childhood (ALSPAC study): an observational cohort study. *The Lancet*, 369(9561), 578-585.

13. Golding, J., et al. (2009). High levels of depressive symptoms in pregnancy with low omega-3 fatty acid intake from fish. *Epidemiology*. 20(4):598-603.
14. United States Geological Survey. (2019). *Environmental and Quality-Control Data Collected by the USGS National Water-Quality Assessment Project for Hormones and Pharmaceuticals in Groundwater Used as a Source of Drinking Water Across the United States, 2013-15.* https://www.usgs.gov/data/environmental-and-quality-control-data-collected-usgs-national-water-quality-assessment. Accessed September 9, 2023.
15. Kosuth, M., et al. (2017). Synthetic Polymer Contamination in Global Drinking Water. *Orb Media.* https://orbmedia.org/invisibles-final-report. Accessed September 9, 2023.
16. Mason, S., et al. (2018). Synthetic Polymer Contamination in Bottled Water. *Frontiers in Chemistry*. 6.
17. Consumer Reports. (2021). Tap Water Testing by Location. https://uploads.guim.co.uk/2021/04/02/Consumer_Reports_Tap_Water_Test_Results_April_2021_(7).pdf. Accessed September 7, 2023.
18. Center for Disease Control. (2022). Germs That Can Contaminate Tap Water. https://www.cdc.gov/healthywater/drinking/contamination/germs.html. Accessed September 7, 2023.
19. Virginia Department of Health. (2018). Cryptosporidiosis and Drinking Water. https://www.vdh.virginia.gov/epidemiology/epidemiology-fact-sheets/cryptosporidiosis-and-drinking-water/#:~:text=Cryptosporidium%20parasites%20get%20into%20surface,like%20form%20of%20the%20parasite. Accessed September 7, 2023.
20. Cox, C. (2017). Trouble in Farm Country: Ag Runoff Fouls Tap Water Across Rural America. *Environmental Working Group*. Retrieved from https://www.ewg.org/tapwater/trouble-in-farm-country.php

21. Campsiano, D. (2023). What Is Cancer Alley? *Verywell Health.* Retrieved from https://www.verywellhealth.com/cancer-alley-5097197#:~:text=Cancer%20Alley%20is%20an%2085,the%20name%20implies%2C%20cancer%20cases. Accessed September 7, 2023.
22. United Stated Environmental Protection Agency. (2024). Key EPA Actions to Address PFAS. *EPA*. Retrieved from https://www.epa.gov/pfas/key-epa-actions-address-pfas
23. Morris, Z., et al. (2011). The answer is 17 years, what is the question: understanding time lags in translational research. *Journal of the Royal Society of Medicine.* 104(12): 510–520.
24. Chang, S. (n.d.). Bottled Water or Tap? Here's Why Your Choice Matters. *Stone Pier Press.* https://stonepierpress.org/goodfoodnews/bottled-water-or-tap#:~:text=Most%20bottled%20water%20is%20actually,and%20Poland%20Spring%2C%20among%20others. Accessed September 9, 2023.
25. Mason, S., et al. (2018). Synthetic Polymer Contamination in Bottled Water. *Frontiers in Chemistry,* 6: 407.
26. Michigan Department of Public Health. Distillation for Home Water Treatment. *Michigan State University.* https://www.baycounty-mi.gov/Docs/CitizenCorps/DistillationForHomeWaterTreatment.pdf. Accessed September 9, 2023.
27. Klepeis, N., et al. (2001). The National Human Activity Pattern Survey (NHAPS): a resource for assessing exposure to environmental pollutants. *Journal of Exposure Science & Environmental Epidemiology.* 11, 231–252.
28. Mitro, S. D., Dodson, R. E., Singla, V., Adamkiewicz, G., Elmi, A. F., Tilly, M. K., & Zota, A. R. (2016). Consumer product chemicals in indoor dust: A quantitative meta-analysis of US studies. *Environmental Science & Technology,* 50(19), 10661-10672.

29. Dodson, R. E., Perovich, L. J., Covaci, A., Van den Eede, N., Ionas, A. C., Dirtu, A. C., ... & Stapleton, H. M. (2012). After the PBDE phase-out: A broad suite of flame retardants in repeat house dust samples from California. *Environmental Science & Technology,* 46(24), 13056-13066.
30. Same as above.
31. Bradman, A., Castorina, R., Sjödin, A., Fenster, L., Jones, R. S., Harley, K. G., ... & Eskenazi, B. (2012). Factors associated with serum polybrominated diphenyl ether (PBDE) levels among school-age children in the CHAMACOS cohort. *Environmental Science & Technology,* 46(13), 7373-7381.
32. Butt, C. M., Congleton, J., Hoffman, K., Fang, M., & Stapleton, H. M. (2014). Metabolites of organophosphate flame retardants and 2-ethylhexyl tetrabromobenzoate in urine from paired mothers and toddlers. *Environmental Science & Technology,* 48(17), 10432-10438.
33. Fang, M., Webster, T. F., & Stapleton, H. M. (2015). Effect-directed analysis of human peroxisome proliferator-activated nuclear receptors (PPARγ1) ligands in indoor dust. *Environmental Science & Technology,* 49(16), 10065-1007.
34. Gosavi, R. A., Knudsen, G. A., Birnbaum, L. S., & Pedersen, L. C. (2013). Mimicking of estradiol binding by flame retardants and their metabolites: A crystallographic analysis. *Environmental Health Perspectives,* 121(10), 1194-1199.
35. Dallaire, R., Dewailly, E., Ayotte, P., Muckle, G., Laliberté, C., Bruneau, S., ... & Jacobson, S. W. (2009). Thyroid function and plasma concentrations of polyhalogenated compounds in Inuit adults. *Environmental Health Perspectives,* 117(9), 1380-1386.
36. Chevrier, J., Harley, K. G., Bradman, A., Sjödin, A., Eskenazi, B., & Holland, N. (2010). Polybrominated diphenyl ether (PBDE) flame retardants and thyroid hormone during pregnancy. *Environmental Health Perspectives,* 118(10), 1444–1449.
37. Boas, M., Main, K. M., & Feldt-Rasmussen, U. (2009). Environmental chemicals and thyroid function: An update. *Current Opinion in Endocrinology, Diabetes and Obesity,* 16(5), 385-391.

38. Talsness, C. E., Shakibaei, M., Kuriyama, S. N., Grande, S. W., Sterner-Kock, A., Schnitker, P., ... & Grote, K. (2005). Ultrastructural changes observed in rat ovaries following in utero and lactational exposure to low doses of a polybrominated flame retardant. *Toxicology Letters,* 157(3), 189-202.
39. Meeker, J. D., & Stapleton, H. M. (2010). House dust concentrations of organophosphate flame retardants in relation to hormone levels and semen quality parameters. *Environmental Health Perspectives,* 118(3), 318-323.
40. Akutsu, K., Takatori, S., Nozawa, S., Yoshiike, M., Nakazawa, H., & Hayakawa, K. (2008). Polybrominated diphenyl ethers in human serum and sperm quality. *Bulletin of Environmental Contamination and Toxicology,* 80(4), 345-350.
41. Deng, X., et al. (2022). Insight into the incredible effects of microwave heating: Driving changes in the structure, properties and functions of macromolecular nutrients in novel food. *Nutrition and Food Science Technology,* 13.
42. Lau, O.-W., & Wong, S.-K. (1996). The migration of plasticizers from cling film into food during microwave heating—Effect of fat content and contact time. *Packaging Technology and Science,* 9(1), 19-27.
43. Lickly, T. D., Lehr, K. M., & Welsh, G. C. (1995). Migration of styrene from polystyrene foam food-contact articles. *Food and Chemical Toxicology,* 33(6), 475-481.
44. Tawfik, M. S., & Huyghebaert, A. (1998). Polystyrene cups and containers: Styrene migration. Food Additives & Contaminants, 15(5), 592-599.
45. Tang, W., Hemm, I., & Eisenbrand, G. (2000). Estimation of human exposure to styrene and ethylbenzene. *Toxicology,* 144(1-3), 39-50.
46. Sati, P. C., Pant, N., Mathur, N., Kumar, M., Saxena, D. K., & Gupta, Y. K. (2011). Pulmonary function and oxidative stress in workers exposed to styrene in plastic factory: Occupational hazards in styrene-exposed plastic factory workers. *Human & Experimental Toxicology,* 30(11), 1743-1750.

47. Qiu, W., Zhao, Y., Yang, M., Farajzadeh, M., Pan, C., Wayne, N. L., & Zhang, B. (2015). Actions of bisphenol A and bisphenol S on the reproductive neuroendocrine system during early development in zebrafish. *Endocrinology,* 157(2), 636-647.
48. Kumar, V., & Gill, K. D. (2009). Aluminium neurotoxicity: Neurobehavioural and oxidative aspects. *Archives of Toxicology,* 83(11), 965-978.
49. Kumar, V., & Gill, K. D. (2014). Oxidative stress and mitochondrial dysfunction in aluminium neurotoxicity and its amelioration: A review. *Neurotoxicology,* 41, 154-166.
50. Flarend, R., Bin, T., Elmore, D., & Hem, S. L. (2001). A preliminary study of the dermal absorption of aluminium from antiperspirants using aluminium-26. *Food and Chemical Toxicology,* 39(2), 163-168.
51. Pineau, A., Fauconneau, B., Sappino, A. P., Deloncle, R., Guillard, O., & Cillard, J. (2012). In vitro study of percutaneous absorption of aluminum from antiperspirants through human skin in the FranzTM diffusion cell. *Journal of Inorganic Biochemistry,* 110, 21-26.
52. Havlicek, J., & Lenochova, P. (2006). The effect of meat consumption on body odor attractiveness. *Chemical Senses,* 31(8), 747-752.
53. Sirotkin, A. V., & Harrath, A. H. (2017). Influence of oil-related environmental pollutants on female reproduction. *Reproductive Toxicology,* 71, 142-145.
54. Avelino, H. (2012, June 19). How to Remove Water Based Nail Polish | Pretty Painted Nails. Pretty Painted Nails.
55. Environmental Working Group. (2009, November 3). *Classroom cleaners release 457 air pollutants: Study findings.* Retrieved from https://static.ewg.org/reports/2009/school_cleaners/EWG-School-Cleaning-Supplies.pdf.
56. Odabasi, M. (2008). Halogenated volatile organic compounds from the use of chlorine-bleach-containing household products. *Environmental Science & Technology,* 42(5), 1445-1451.

57. Naz, K., Shah, F. A., Liaqat, I., Rehman, F., Shah, S. T. A., Ahmad, F., & Ullah, S. (2014). Pistacia chinensis: A potent ameliorator of CCl4 induced lung and thyroid toxicity in rat model. *BioMed Research International*, 2014.
58. U.S. Environmental Protection Agency. (n.d.). Hazard Summary, Glycol Ethers (2-Butoxyethanol): Uses, sources and potential exposure, acute and chronic health hazard information, and more). Retrieved from https://www.epa.gov/sites/default/files/2016-09/documents/glycol-ethers.pdf
59. Agency for Toxic Substances and Disease Registry. (1999). ToxFAQsTM for 2-Butoxyethanol and 2-Butoxyethanol Acetate. Retrieved from https://www.atsdr.cdc.gov/toxfaqs/tfacts118.pdf. Accessed September 9, 2023.
60. Grün, F., & Blumberg, B. (2009). Endocrine disrupters as obesogens. *Molecular and Cellular Endocrinology*, 304(1-2), 19-29.
61. Melin, V., et al. (2014). Exposure to common quaternary ammonium disinfectants decreases fertility in mice. *Reproductive Toxicology*, 50:163-70.
62. Shafik, A. (1993). Effect of different types of textile fabric on spermatogenesis: an experimental study. *Urology Research and Practice*, 21(5):367-70.
63. Shafik, A. (1992). Contraceptive efficacy of polyester-induced azoospermia in normal men. *Contraception*, 45(5):439-51.

Chapter 10: Addressing Mold Exposures and Mold in Your Body

1. Surviving Mold. (n.d.). The Shoemaker Protocol Visual Contrast Sensitivity Test (VCS). Retrieved from https://www.survivingmold.com/resources-for-patients/diagnosis/visual-contrast-sensitivity-vcs
2. Vradelis, S., Kalaitzakis, E., Sharifi, Y., et al. (2009). Addition of senna improves quality of colonoscopy preparation with magnesium citrate. *World Journal of Gastroenterology*, 15(14), 1759-1763.

3. Guarize, L., Costa, J. C., Dutra, L. B., Mendes, R. F., Lima, I. V., & Scio, E. (2012). Anti-inflammatory, laxative and intestinal motility effects of Senna macranthera leaves. *Natural Product Research,* 26(4), 331-343.
4. Lai, Y., et al. (2022). Mycotoxins binder supplementation alleviates aflatoxin B1 toxic effects on the immune response and intestinal barrier function in broilers. *Poultry Science,* 101(3):101683.
5. Hope, J. (2013). A review of the mechanism of injury and treatment approaches for illness resulting from exposure to water-damaged buildings, mold, and mycotoxins. *The Scientific World Journal,* 2013, 767482.
6. Wang, P., Afriyie-Gyawu, E., Tang, Y., et al. (2008). NovaSil clay intervention in Ghanaians at high risk for aflatoxicosis: II. Reduction in biomarkers of aflatoxin exposure in blood and urine. *Food Additives & Contaminants Part A: Chemistry, Analysis, Control, Exposure & Risk Assessment,* 25(5), 622-634.
7. Phillips, T. D., Afriyie-Gyawu, E., Williams, J., et al. (2008). Reducing human exposure to aflatoxin through the use of clay: A review. *Food Additives & Contaminants Part A: Chemistry, Analysis, Control, Exposure & Risk Assessment,* 25(2), 134-145.
8. Gross-Steinmeyer, K., & Eaton, D. L. (2012). Dietary modulation of the biotransformation and genotoxicity of aflatoxin B(1). *Toxicology,* 299(2-3), 69-79.
9. Decker, W. J., & Corby, D. G. (1980). Activated charcoal adsorbs aflatoxin B1. Veterinary and Human Toxicology, 22(6), 388-389.
10. Boudergue, C., Burel, C., Dragacci, S., et al. (2009). Review of mycotoxin-detoxifying agents used as feed additives: Mode of action, efficacy and feed/food safety. *EFSA Support Publications,* 6(9).
11. Vetvicka, V. (2014). Effects of β-glucan on some environmental toxins: An overview. *Biomedical Papers of the Medical Faculty of the University Palacký, Olomouc, Czech Republic,* 158(1), 1-4.

12. Dvorák, M. (1989). Schopnost bentonitu a prírodního zeolitu adsorbovat aflatoxin z tekutých prostredí [Ability of bentonite and natural zeolite to adsorb aflatoxin from liquid media]. *Veterinární Medicína (Praha),* 34(5), 307-316.
13. Pattar, J., Shridhar, N. B., Suhasini, K., et al. (2020). Protective role of diatomaceous earth (DAE) on combined mycotoxicosis of aflatoxin B1 and ochratoxin A in coloured broiler (RAJA II) chickens. *Journal of Entomology and Zoology Studies,* 8(2), 1424-1429.
14. Murthy, T. N. K., Reddy, B. N., & Devegowda, G. (2002). Evaluation of glucomannan for its adsorbing ability of aflatoxin B1 and T-2 toxin in the gastrointestinal tract of broiler chickens. *Mycotoxin Research,* 18(1), 20–23.
15. Istiqomah, L., Damayanti, E., Arisnandhy, D., et al. (2019). Saccharomyces cerevisiae B18 as antifungal and aflatoxin binder in vitro. In *AIP Conference Proceedings* 2099 (p. 020009).
16. Kosztik, J., Mörtl, M., Székács, A., Kukolya, J., & Bata-Vidács, I. (2020). Aflatoxin B1 and sterigmatocystin binding potential of lactobacilli. *Toxins,* 12(12), 756.
17. De Jesus, C. L., Bartley, A., Welch, A. Z., & Berry, J. P. (2017). High incidence and levels of ochratoxin A in wines sourced from the United States. *Toxins,* 10(1), 1.
18. Joannis-Cassan, C., Tozlovanu, M., Hadjeba-Medjdoub, K., et al. (2011). Zearalenone, aflatoxin B1, and ochratoxin A by yeast-based products: A method for quantification of adsorption performance. *Journal of Food Protection,* 74(7), 1175-1185.
19. Kerkadi, A., Barriault, C., Marquardt, R. R., et al. (1999). Cholestyramine protection against ochratoxin A toxicity: Role of ochratoxin A sorption by the resin and bile acid enterohepatic circulation. *Journal of Food Protection,* 62(12), 1461-1465.
20. Armando, M. R., Pizzolitto, R. P., Dogi, C. A., et al. (2012). Adsorption of ochratoxin A and zearalenone by potential probiotic Saccharomyces cerevisiae strains and its relation with cell wall thickness. *Journal of Applied Microbiology,* 113(2), 256-264.

21. Karami-Osboo, R., Maham, M., & Nasrollahzadeh, M. (2020). Synthesised magnetic nano-zeolite as a mycotoxins binder to reduce the toxicity of aflatoxins, zearalenone, ochratoxin A, and deoxynivalenol in barley. *IET Nanobiotechnology*, 14(7), 623-627.
22. Chlebicz, A., & Śliżewska, K. (2020). In vitro detoxification of aflatoxin B1, deoxynivalenol, fumonisins, T-2 toxin and zearalenone by probiotic bacteria from genus Lactobacillus and Saccharomyces cerevisiae yeast. *Probiotics and Antimicrobial Proteins*, 12(1), 289-301.
23. Karami-Osboo, R., Maham, M., & Nasrollahzadeh, M. (2020). Synthesised magnetic nano-zeolite as a mycotoxins binder to reduce the toxicity of aflatoxins, zearalenone, ochratoxin A, and deoxynivalenol in barley. *IET Nanobiotechnology*, 14(7), 623-627.
24. Bertero, A., Fossati, P., Tedesco, D. E. A., & Caloni, F. (2020). Beauvericin and Enniatins: In Vitro Intestinal Effects. *Toxins* (Basel), 12(11), 686.
25. Niderkorn, V., Morgavi, D., Aboab, B., Lemaire, M., & Boudra, H. (2009). Cell wall component and mycotoxin moieties involved in the binding of fumonisin B1 and B2 by lactic acid bacteria. *Journal of Applied Microbiology*, 106, 977-985.
26. Kamle, M., Mahato, D. K., Gupta, A., et al. (2022). Citrinin mycotoxin contamination in food and feed: impact on agriculture, human health, and detection and management strategies. *Toxins* (Basel), 14(2), 85.
27. Ioi, J. D., Zhou, T., Tsao, R., & Marcone, F. M. (2017). Mitigation of patulin in fresh and processed foods and beverages. *Toxins* (Basel), 9(5), 157.
28. Novak, M., & Vetvicka, V. (2008). B-glucans, history, and the present: Immunomodulatory aspects and mechanisms of action. *Journal of Immunotoxicology*, 5(1), 47-57.
29. Oporto, C. I., Villarroel, C. A., Tapia, S. M., García, V., & Cubillos, F. A. (2019). Distinct transcriptional changes in response to patulin underlie toxin biosorption differences in Saccharomyces cerevisiae. *Toxins* (Basel), 11(7), 400.

30. Moosavi, M. (2017). Bentonite clay as a natural remedy: A brief review. Iranian Journal of Public Health, 46(9), 1176-1183.
31. Zhou, X., Zhao, A., Goping, G., & Hirszel, P. (2000). Gliotoxin-induced cytotoxicity proceeds via apoptosis and is mediated by caspases and reactive oxygen species in LLC-PK1 cells. *Toxicological Sciences*, 54(1), 194-202.
32. Chugh, R. M., et al. (2022). Fungal Mushrooms: A Natural Compound With Therapeutic Applications. Frontiers in Pharmacology, 13: 925387.
33. Batista, L. R., et al. (2009). Ochratoxin A in coffee beans (Coffea arabica L.) processed by dry and wet methods. *Food Control*, 20 (9), 784-790.
34. Benites, A. J., et al. (2017). Occurrence of ochratoxin A in roasted coffee samples commercialized in Portugal. *Food Control*, 73B, 1223- 1228.
35. Attiya, W. A., et al. (2021). Prevalence of toxigenic fungi and mycotoxins in Arabic coffee (Coffea arabica): Protective role of traditional coffee roasting, brewing and bacterial volatiles. *PLOS ONE*, 16(10): e0259302.

Chapter 11: Supporting Mitochondrial Function for Healthy Organs

1. Zhang, D., et al. (2017). Mitochondria in oocyte aging: current understanding. *Facts, Views, and Visions*, 9(1): 29–38.
2. Naviaux, R. (2019). Metabolic features and regulation of the healing cycle—A new model for chronic disease pathogenesis and treatment. *Mitochondrion*, 46, 278-297.
3. Same as above.
4. Velarde, M. (2014). Mitochondrial and sex steroid hormone crosstalk during aging. *Longevity & Healthspan*, 3: 2.

5. Podolak, A., et al. (2022). The Role of Mitochondria in Human Fertility and Early Embryo Development: What Can We Learn for Clinical Application of Assessing and Improving Mitochondrial DNA? *Cells,* 11(5): 797.
6. Cecchino, G. N. (2018). The role of mitochondrial activity in female fertility and assisted reproductive technologies: overview and current insights. *Reproductive Biomedicine Online,* 36(6), 686-697.
7. Chiang, J., et al. (2020). Mitochondria in Ovarian Aging and Reproductive Longevity. *Ageing Research Reviews,* 63, 101168.
8. Dezest, M., et al. (2017). Oxidative damage and impairment of protein quality control systems in keratinocytes exposed to a volatile organic compounds cocktail. *Scientific Reports,* 7: 10707.
9. Balali-Mood, M., et al. (2021). Toxic Mechanisms of Five Heavy Metals: Mercury, Lead, Chromium, Cadmium, and Arsenic. *Frontiers in Pharmacology,* 12.
10. Cheng, H., et al. (2021). Mechanisms of Metal-Induced Mitochondrial Dysfunction in Neurological Disorders. *Toxics,* 9(6), 142.
11. Zhang, J., et al. (2022). Lead Disrupts Mitochondrial Morphology and Function through Induction of ER Stress in Model of Neurotoxicity. *International Journal of Molecular Sciences,* 23(19):11435.
12. Cheng, H., et al. (2021). Mechanisms of Metal-Induced Mitochondrial Dysfunction in Neurological Disorders. *Toxics,* 9(6), 142.
13. Janik-Karpinska, E., et al. (2023). Mitochondrial Damage Induced by T-2 Mycotoxin on Human Skin—Fibroblast Hs68 Cell Line. *Molecules,* 28(5): 2408.
14. Strilbyska, O. M., et al. (2022). The effects of low-toxic herbicide Roundup and glyphosate on mitochondria. *EXCLI Journal,* 21: 183–196.
15. Sharma, B., et al. (2014). Biomedical Implications of Heavy Metals Induced Imbalances in Redox Systems. *BioMed Research International,* 2014.

16. Filler, K., et al. (2014). Association of mitochondrial dysfunction and fatigue: A review of the literature. *BBA Clinical,* 1: 12–23.
17. Schmitt, K., Grimm, A., Dallmann, R., & et al. (2018). Circadian control of DRP1 activity regulates mitochondrial dynamics and bioenergetics. *Cell Metabolism,* 27(3), 657-666.e5.
18. Rodrigues, N. R., Macedo, G. E., Martins, I. K., & et al. (2018). Short-term sleep deprivation with exposure to nocturnal light alters mitochondrial bioenergetics in Drosophila. *Free Radical Biology & Medicine,* 120, 395-406.
19. Picard, M., & McEwen, B. S. (2018). Psychological stress and mitochondria: A systematic review. *Psychosomatic Medicine,* 80(2), 141-153.
20. Memme, J., et al. (2019). Exercise and mitochondrial health. *The Journal of Physiology,* 5(3): 803-817.
21. Kyriazis, I., et al. (2022). The impact of diet upon mitochondrial physiology (Review). *International Journal of Molecular Medicine,* 50(5).
22. Parson, V. & Ramsay, I. (1968). Thyroid and adrenal relationships. *Postgraduate Medicine Journal,* 44(511): 377–384.
23. Pizzorno, J. (2014). Mitochondria—Fundamental to Life and Health. *Integrative Medicine: A Clinician's Journal,* 13(2): 8–15.
24. McMackin, C. J., Widlansky, M. E., Hamburg, N. M., & et al. (2007). Effect of combined treatment with alpha-Lipoic acid and acetyl-L-carnitine on vascular function and blood pressure in patients with coronary artery disease. *Journal of Clinical Hypertension (Greenwich),* 9(4), 249–255.
25. Lagouge, M., Argmann, C., Gerhart-Hines, Z., & et al. (2006). Resveratrol improves mitochondrial function and protects against metabolic disease by activating SIRT1 and PGC-1α. *Cell,* 127(6), 1109–1122.
26. Timmers, S., Konings, E., Bilet, L., & et al. (2011). Calorie restriction-like effects of 30 days of resveratrol supplementation on energy metabolism and metabolic profile in obese humans. *Cell Metabolism,* 14(5), 612–622.

27. Kelly, N. A., Ford, M. P., Standaert, D. G., & et al. (2014). Novel, high-intensity exercise prescription improves muscle mass, mitochondrial function, and physical capacity in individuals with Parkinson's disease. *Journal of Applied Physiology*, 1985(Jan).

Chapter 12: The Pillar of Liver Detoxification

1. Kalra, A., et al. (2023). Physiology, Liver. Stat Pearls.
2. Samsel, A. & Seneff, S. (2013). Glyphosate, pathways to modern diseases II: Celiac sprue and gluten intolerance. Interdisciplinary *Toxicology*, 6(4):159-84.
3. Jancova, P., et al. (2010). Phase II Drug Metabolizing Enzymes. *Biomed Pap Med Fac Univ Palacky Olomouc Czech Repub*, 154(2):103–116.
4. Lobos, P. & Regulska-Ilow, B. (2023). Link between methyl nutrients and the DNA methylation process in the course of selected diseases in adults. *Roczniki Państwowego Zakładu Higieny*, 72(2):123-136.
5. Moll, S., & Varga, E. A. (2015). Homocysteine and MTHFR mutations. *Circulation*, 132(1), e6–e9.
6. Sibani, S., et al. (2000). Characterization of six novel mutations in the methylenetetrahydrofolate reductase (MTHFR) gene in patients with homocystinuria. *Human Mutation*, 15(3):280-7.
7. Silvagno, F., et al. (2020). The Role of Glutathione in Protecting against the Severe Inflammatory Response Triggered by COVID-19. *Antioxidants*, 9(7): 624.
8. Hodges, R. & Minich, D. (2015). Modulation of Metabolic Detoxification Pathways Using Foods and Food-Derived Components: A Scientific Review with Clinical Application. *Nutrition and Metabolism*, 2015: 760689.
9. Same as above.
10. Phang-Lyn, S. & Llerena, V. (2023). Biochemistry, Biotransformation. *StatPearls*.

11. Swain, M. (2006). Fatigue in liver disease: Pathophysiology and clinical management. *Canadian Journal of Gastroenterology*, 20(3): 181–188.
12. Azhari, H. & Swain, M. (2018). Role of Peripheral Inflammation in Hepatic Encephalopathy. *Journal of Clinical and Experimental Hepatology*, 8(3): 281–285.
13. Ziem, G. & McTamney, J. (1997). Profile of patients with chemical injury and sensitivity. *Environmental Health Perspectives*, 105(Suppl 2): 417–436.
14. Green, C. & Hodson, L. (2014). The Influence of Dietary Fat on Liver Fat Accumulation. *Nutrients*, 6(11): 5018–5033.
15. Patrushev, N. B., et al. (2010). Conservative treatment of patients with varicose esophagus veins cirrhosis. *Eksp Klin Gastroenterology Journal*, (11):40-5.
16. Galati, G., et al. (2014). Haemorrhoidal disease in severe portal hypertension: a combined approach with transjugular intrahepatic portosystemic shunt (TIPS) and transanal haemorrhoidal dearterialization (THD). *Archives of Medical Science*, 10(1): 195–196.
17. Manenti, G., Picchi, E., Castrignanò, A., Muto, M., Nezzo, M., & Floris, R. (2016). Liver lipoma: A case report. *BJR Case Reports*, 3(2), 20150467.
18. Kwon, C., et al. (2020). Liver-associated patterns as anger syndromes in traditional Chinese medicine: A preliminary literature review with theoretical framework based on the World Health Organization standards of terminologies and pattern diagnosis standards. *European Journal of Integrative Medicine*, 36.
19. Palmisano, B., et al. (2018). Estrogens in the Regulation of Liver Lipid Metabolism. *Advances in Experimental Medicine and Biology*, 1043: 227–256.
20. Koulaouzidis, A., et al. (2007). Skin manifestations of liver diseases. *Annals of Hepatology*, 6(3), 181-184.
21. Sanglodkar, U., et al. (2018). Cellulitis in liver cirrhosis – a series of 25 cases from southern India. *Clinical and Experimental Hepatology*, 4(3): 201–204.

22. Aneni, E., et al. (2015). Blood pressure is associated with the presence and severity of nonalcoholic fatty liver disease across the spectrum of cardiometabolic risk. *Journal of Hypertension,* 33(6):1207-14.
23. Immel, J. (n.d.). Cholagogues - Food and Herb List. Joyful Belly. Retrieved from https://www.joyfulbelly.com/Ayurveda/herbal-action/cholagogue. Accessed September 8, 2023.
24. Kieffer, D. A., Martin, R. J., & Adams, S. H. (2016). Impact of dietary fibers on nutrient management and detoxification organs: Gut, liver, and kidneys. *Advances in Nutrition,* 7(6), 1111-1121.

Chapter 13: Restoring Gut Harmony

1. Sender, R., et al. (2016). Revised Estimates for the Number of Human and Bacteria Cells in the Body. *PLOS Biology,* 14(8): e1002533.
2. Wiertsema, S., et al. (2021). The Interplay between the Gut Microbiome and the Immune System in the Context of Infectious Diseases throughout Life and the Role of Nutrition in Optimizing Treatment Strategies. *Nutrients,* 13(3): 886.
3. Terry, N. & Margolis, K. G. (2017). Serotonergic Mechanisms Regulating the GI Tract: Experimental Evidence and Therapeutic Relevance. *Handbook of Experimental Pharmacology,* 239: 319–342.
4. Rowland, I., et al. (2018). Gut microbiota functions: metabolism of nutrients and other food components. *European Journal of Nutrition,* 57(1): 1–24.
5. Kellie, F. (2017). Vitamin K supplementation during pregnancy for improving outcomes. *Cochrane Database of Systematic Reviews,* (6): CD010920.
6. De Pessemier, B., et al. (2021). Gut–Skin Axis: Current Knowledge of the Interrelationship between Microbial Dysbiosis and Skin Conditions. *Microorganisms,* 9(2): 353.
7. Salazar, A., et al. (2022). Gut-bladder axis enters the stage: Implication for recurrent urinary tract infections. *Cell Host Microbe,* 30(8): 1066–1069.

8. Kobayashi, H. (2023). Gut and reproductive tract microbiota: Insights into the pathogenesis of endometriosis (Review). *Biomedical Reports,* 19(1): 43.
9. Centers for Disease Control and Prevention. (2021). Outpatient Antibiotic Prescriptions — United States, 2021. Retrieved from https://archive.cdc.gov/#/details?url=https://www.cdc.gov/antibiotic-use/data/report-2021.html
10. National Center for Health Statistics. (2024). Total Cesarean deliveries by race: United States, 2020-2022 Average. March of Dimes. Retrieved from https://www.marchofdimes.org/peristats/
11. Duong, Q., et al. (2022). Antibiotic exposure and adverse long-term health outcomes in children: A systematic review and meta-analysis. *Journal of Infection,* 85(3): 213-300
12. Harvard T.H. Chan. (n.d.). "The Microbiome." The Nutrition Source. Retrieved from https://nutritionsource.hsph.harvard.edu/microbiome/#:~:text=If%20one%20does%20not%20have,in%20a%20lower%20acidic%20environment.
13. Kaliannan, K., et al. (2015). A host-microbiome interaction mediates the opposing effects of omega-6 and omega-3 fatty acids on metabolic endotoxemia. *Scientific Reports,* 5:11276.
14. Guilliams, T. & Drake, L. (2020). Meal-Time Supplementation with Betaine HCl for Functional Hypochlorhydria: What is the Evidence? *Integrative Medicine: A Clinician's Journal,* 19(1): 32–36.
15. Jamal, M., et al. (2018). Bacterial biofilm and associated infections. *Journal of Chinese Medicine Association,* 8(1): 7-11.
16. Man, A., et al. (2017). New perspectives on the nutritional factors influencing growth rate of Candida albicans in diabetics. An in vitro study. *Memorias Do Instituto Oswaldo Cruz,* 112(9): 587–592.
17. Mottaghi, B., et al. (2021). Candida colonization of the esophagus and gastric mucosa; a comparison of patients taking proton pump inhibitors and those taking histamine receptor antagonist drugs. *Gastroenterology and Hepatology from Bed to Bench,* 14(4): 349–355.

18. Akimoto-Gunther, L., et al. (2016). Highlights Regarding Host Predisposing Factors to Recurrent Vulvovaginal Candidiasis: Chronic Stress and Reduced Antioxidant Capacity. *PLOS ONE,* 11(7): e0158870.
19. Aminzadeh, A., et al. (2016). Frequency of Candidiasis and Colonization of Candida albicans in Relation to Oral Contraceptive Pills. *Iranian Red Crescent Medical Journal,* 18(10): e38909.
20. National Organization for Rare Disorders. (n.d.). Systemic candidiasis. Retrieved from https://rarediseases.org/gard-rare-disease/systemic-candidiasis/
21. University of Colorado. (n.d.). Diabetes and Birth Control. Retrieved from https://obgyn.coloradowomenshealth.com/health-info/birth-control/medical-conditions-birth-control/diabetes
22. Kumwenda, P., et al. (2022). Estrogen promotes innate immune evasion of Candida albicans through inactivation of the alternative complement system. *Cell Reports,* 38(1):110183.
23. Ullrich, I. H., et al. (1985). Effect of low-carbohydrate diets high in either fat or protein on thyroid function, plasma insulin, glucose, and triglycerides in healthy young adults. *Journal of the American College of Nutrition,* 4(4):451-459.
24. Barrea, L., et al. (2023). Effects of very low-calorie ketogenic diet on hypothalamic–pituitary–adrenal axis and renin–angiotensin–aldosterone system. *Journal of Endocrinological Investigation,* 46: 1509–1520.
25. Ferreira, L. F., et al. (2014). Parasite Findings in Archeological Remains: a paleogeographic view. *Foundations of Paleoparasitology,* 307-339.
26. Hotez, P. & Herricks, J. (2015). "One Million Deaths by Parasites." *PLOS Blogs, Speaking of Medicine and Health.*
27. Kranjcić-Zec, I., et al. (2004). The role of parasites and fungi in secondary infertility. *Medicinski Pregled,* 57(1-2):30-2.
28. Macer, M. L. & Taylor, H. S. (2013). Endometriosis and Infertility: A review of the pathogenesis and treatment of endometriosis-associated infertility. *Obstetrics and Gynecology Clinics of North America,* 39(4): 535–549.

29. Reipen, J., et al. (2012). Peritoneal enterobiasis causing endometriosis-like symptoms. *Clinical and Experimental Obstetrics & Gynecology*, 39(3):379-81.
30. "Bumping Iron No Cure for Hookworms." (2006). Science. https://www.science.org/content/article/bumping-iron-no-cure-hookworms. Accessed August 1, 2023.
31. Zaidi, A., et al. (2017). Leishmania and its quest for iron: An update and overview. *Molecular and Biochemical Parasitology*, 211:15-25.
32. Prueksapanich, P., et al. (2018). Liver Fluke-Associated Biliary Tract Cancer. *Gut and Liver*, 12(3):236-245.
33. Choi, T. & Wong, J. (1984). Severe acute pancreatitis caused by parasites in the common bile duct. *American Journal of Tropical Medicine and Hygiene*, 87(5):211-4.
34. Deftly, C., et al. (2013). Demodex folliculorum: A parasite infection mimicking skin cancer. *Journal of Plastic, Reconstructive & Aesthetic Surgery*, 6(2), 289-290.
35. Pires, M., et al. (2019). The impact of leishmaniasis on mental health and psychosocial well-being: A systematic review. *PLOS ONE*, 14(10): e0223313.
36. Potts, R., et al. (2016). Mast cells and histamine alter intestinal permeability during malaria parasite infection. *Immunobiology*, 221(3): 468–474.
37. Flegr, J. & Horáček, J. (2019). Negative Effects of Latent Toxoplasmosis on Mental Health. *Frontiers of Psychiatry*, 10: 1012.
38. United Network for Organ Sharing. (2017). Guidance regarding donor Toxoplasma screening and organ acceptance. Retrieved from https://unos.org/news/guidance-regarding-donor-toxoplasma-screening-and-organ-acceptance/
39. Al-Malki, E. (2021). Toxoplasmosis: stages of the protozoan life cycle and risk assessment in humans and animals for an enhanced awareness and an improved socio-economic status. *Saudi Journal of Biological Sciences*, 28(1): 962–969.
40. Jarroll, E. L., et al. (1981). Effect of chlorine on Giardia lamblia cyst viability. *Applied and Environmental Microbiology*, 41(2):483-7.

41. "Tapeworm Infection." (2022). Cleveland Clinic. https://my.clevelandclinic.org/health/diseases/23950-tapeworm-infection
42. Pham, K., et al. (2023). Effects of helminths and anthelmintic treatment on cardiometabolic diseases and risk factors: A systematic review. *PLOS Neglected Tropical Diseases,* 17(2): e0011022.
43. Sures, B., Nachev, M., Selbach, C. et al. (2017). Parasite responses to pollution: what we know and where we go in 'Environmental Parasitology.' *Parasites & Vectors,* 10, 65.
44. Yen Nhi, T. T., et al. (2013). Use of cestodes as indicator of heavy-metal pollution. Experimental Parasitology, 133(1): 75-79.
45. Patient Centered Care Advocacy Group. (2016). "Lyme Bacteria Hides Inside Parasitic Worms, Causing Chronic Brain Diseases." *PR Newswire.* https://www.prnewswire.com/news-releases/lyme-bacteria-hides-inside-parasitic-worms-causing-chronic-brain-diseases-300270742.html
46. Omarova, A., et al. (2018). Protozoan Parasites in Drinking Water: A System Approach for Improved Water, Sanitation and Hygiene in Developing Countries. *International Journal of Environmental Research and Public Health,* 15(3): 495.
47. Virginia Department of Health. (2018). Cryptosporidiosis and Drinking Water. https://www.vdh.virginia.gov/epidemiology/epidemiology-fact-sheets/cryptosporidiosis-and-drinking-water/#:~:text=Cryptosporidium%20parasites%20get%20into%20surface,like%20form%20of%20the%20parasite. Accessed September 7, 2023.
48. Levine, G. I. (1991). Sexually transmitted parasitic diseases. *Journal of Primary Care & Community Health,* 18(1):101-28.
49. Shelton, A. (2004). Sexually Transmitted Parasitic Diseases. Clinics in Colon and Rectal Surgery, 17(4): 231-234
50. Center for Disease Control. (n.d.) What Causes Parasitic Diseases. *CDC.* Retrieved from https://www.cdc.gov/parasites/
51. Institute of Medicine (US) Committee on the Economics of Antimalarial Drugs. (2004). Saving Lives, Buying Time: Economics of Malaria Drugs in an Age of Resistance. Washington (DC): *National Academies Press.*

52. Atambay, M., et al. (2007). The frequency of intestinal parasites and head lice among students of the Akşemsettin Primary School for Deaf Students. *Türkiye Parazitoloji Dergisi,* 31(1):62-5.
53. Saetre, K., et al. (2018). Congenital Babesiosis After Maternal Infection With Borrelia burgdorferi and Babesia microti. *Journal of the Pediatric Infectious Diseases Society,* 7(1):e1-e5.
54. Loke, Y. W. (1982). Transmission of parasites across the placenta. Advanced Parasitology, 21:155-228.
55. McAuley, J. (2014). Congenital Toxoplasmosis. *Journal of the Pediatric Infectious Diseases Society,* 3 Suppl 1(Suppl 1):S30-5.
56. Umbrello, G., et al. (2021). Hookworm infection in infants: a case report and review of literature. *Italian Journal of Pediatrics,* 47(1):26.
57. Kutty, P. K. (2014). Breastfeeding and risk of parasitic infection-a review. *Asian Pacific Journal of Tropical Biomedicine,* 4(11), 847-858.

Chapter 14: Hypothyroidism and Revitalizing Function

1. Wyne, K. L., et al. (2022). Hypothyroidism Prevalence in the United States: A Retrospective Study Combining National Health and Nutrition Examination Survey and Claims Data, 2009–2019. *Journal of Endocrine Society,* 7(1): bvac172.
2. Chiovato, L., et al. (2019). Hypothyroidism in Context: Where We've Been and Where We're Going. *Advances in Therapy,* 36(Suppl 2): 47–58.
3. Chen, A., et al. (2013). Thyroid Hormones in Relation to Lead, Mercury, and Cadmium Exposure in the National Health and Nutrition Examination Survey, 2007–2008. *Environmental Health Perspectives,* 121(2): 181–186.
4. Pamphlett, R., et al. (2021). Mercury in the human thyroid gland: Potential implications for thyroid cancer, autoimmune thyroiditis, and hypothyroidism. *PLOS ONE,* 16(2): e0246748.
5. Gallagher, C., et al. (2012). Mercury and thyroid autoantibodies in U.S. women, NHANES 2007–2008. Environmental International, 40, 39-43.

6. Soldin, O., et al. (2013). Thyroid Hormones and Methylmercury Toxicity. *Biological Trace Element Research,* 126(0): 1–12.
7. Zhu, E., et al. (2000). The endocrine disruptive effects of mercury. *Environmental Health and Preventative Medicine,* 4(4): 174–183.
8. De Freitas Cayres, L. S., et al. (2021). Detection of Alterations in the Gut Microbiota and Intestinal Permeability in Patients With Hashimoto Thyroiditis. *Frontiers in Immunology,* 5(12), 579140.
9. Brimhall, J. (2012). Toxic Halogens in our Food and Water Supply. Retrieved from https://www.brimhall.com/p-253-september-24-puzzle-piece-toxic-halogens-in-our-food-and-water-supply.aspx.
10. Eom, Y. S., et al. (2022). Links between Thyroid Disorders and Glucose Homeostasis. *Diabetes and Metabolism Journal,* 46(2): 239–256.
11. Iacovides, S., et al. (2022). Could the ketogenic diet induce a shift in thyroid function and support a metabolic advantage in healthy participants? A pilot randomized-controlled-crossover trial. *PLOS ONE,* 17(6): e0269440.
12. Myers, I. (2022). "This cancer-causing chemical may be lurking in your bread." *Environmental Working Group.* Retrieved from https://www.ewg.org/news-insights/news/2022/05/cancer-causing-chemical-may-be-lurking-your-bread
13. Lv, C., et al. (2021). High Iodine Induces the Proliferation of Papillary and Anaplastic Thyroid Cancer Cells via AKT/Wee1/CDK1 Axis. *Frontiers in Oncology,* 11.
14. Panth, P., et al. (2019). A Review of Iodine Status of Women of Reproductive Age in the USA. *Biological Trace Element Research,*188, 208–220.
15. Same as above.
16. Tinggi, U. (2008). Selenium: its role as antioxidant in human health. *Environmental Health and Preventative Medicine,* 13(2): 102–108.
17. Kang, D., et al. (2020). The role of selenium metabolism and selenoproteins in cartilage homeostasis and arthropathies. *Experimental and Molecular Medicine,* 52(8): 1198–1208.

18. Duarte Tortelly Costa, V., et al. (2018). The Relevance of Selenium to Alopecias. International Journal of Trichology, 10(2): 92–93.
19. Iorizzo, M., et al. (2022). Leukonychia: What Can White Nails Tell Us? *American Journal of Clinical Dermatology*, 23(2): 177–193.
20. Van Zuuren, E., et al. (2014). Selenium Supplementation for Hashimoto's Thyroiditis: Summary of a Cochrane Systematic Review. *European Thyroid Journal*, 3(1): 25–31.
21. Institute of Medicine. (1997). Dietary Reference Intakes for Calcium, Phosphorus, Magnesium, Vitamin D, and Fluoride. Washington, DC: *National Academy Press*.
22. Gatea, M. (2021). Ending the Autoimmune Epidemic With Natural Functional Medicine. *Fullscript*. Web.
23. Ihnatowicz, P., et al. (2021). The importance of gluten exclusion in the management of Hashimoto's thyroiditis. *Annals of Agricultural and Environmental Medicine*, 28(4):558-568.

Chapter 15: Crucial Nutrient Replenishment

1. Baerwald, A. R. & Pierson, R. A. (2010). Ovarian Follicular Development During the Use of Oral Contraception: A Review. *Canadian Institutes of Health Research*, 26(1): 19–24.
2. Palmery, M., et al. (2013). Oral contraceptives and changes in nutritional requirements. *European Review for Medical and Pharmacological Sciences*, 17(13):1804-13.
3. Same as above.
4. Crider, K. S., Bailey, L. B., & Berry, R. J. (2011). Folic acid food fortification-its history, effect, concerns, and future directions [Conference presentation]. *Nutrients*, 3(3), 370-384.
5. Greenberg, J., et al. (2011). Folic Acid Supplementation and Pregnancy: More Than Just Neural Tube Defect Prevention. *Reviews in Obstetrics & Gynecology*, 4(2): 52–59.
6. Chavarro, J. E., et al. (2008). Use of multivitamins, intake of B vitamins and risk of ovulatory infertility. *Fertility and Sterility*, 89(3): 668–676.

7. "Vitamin B6 and Fertility." (n.d.) Impryl. Retrieved from https://imprylusa.com/nutrition/b6-and-fertility/.
8. "Aiding conception with supplements." (2015). Mums in the Wood. Retrieved from https://mumsinthewood.com/conceive-them/aiding-conception-with-supplements/
9. Chavarro, J. E., et al. (2008). Use of multivitamins, intake of B vitamins and risk of ovulatory infertility. *Fertility and Sterility,* 89(3): 668–676.
10. Shane, B. & Stokstad, E. L. (1985). Vitamin B12-folate interrelationships. *Annual Review of Nutrition,* 5:115-41.
11. Cuciureanu, M. D. & Vink, R. (2011). Magnesium and stress. Adelaide (AU): *University of Adelaide Press.*
12. Lopresti, A. (2020) The Effects of Psychological and Environmental Stress on Micronutrient Concentrations in the Body: A Review of the Evidence. *Advances in Nutrition,* 11(1): 103–112.
13. "The vicious cycle of magnesium deficiency and stress." (2022). Nature's Source. Retrieved from https://www.natures-source.com/en-us/blogs/news/the-vicious-cycle-of-magnesium-deficiency-and-stress.
14. Rivlin, R. S. (1994). Magnesium deficiency and alcohol intake: mechanisms, clinical significance and possible relation to cancer development (a review). *Journal of the American College of Nutrition,* 13(5):416-23.
15. Simopoulos, A. P. (2022). The importance of the ratio of omega-6/omega-3 essential fatty acids. *Biomedicine & Pharmacotherapy,* 56(8):365-79.
16. Ouladsahebmadarek, E., et al. (2014). Hormonal and metabolic effects of polyunsaturated fatty acid (omega-3) on polycystic ovary syndrome induced rats under diet. *Iranian Journal of Basic Medical Sciences,* 17(2): 123–127.
17. Same as above.
18. Sinha, S., et al. (2023). The Effect of Omega-3 Fatty Acids on Insulin Resistance. *Life,* 13(6), 1322.

19. Jouris, K. B., et al. (2011). The Effect of Omega-3 Fatty Acid Supplementation on the Inflammatory Response to eccentric strength exercise. *Journal of Sports Science & Medicine,* 10(3): 432–438.
20. Saldeen, P. & Saldeen, T. (2004). Women and omega-3 Fatty acids. *Obstetrical & Gynecological Survey,* 59(10):722-30.
21. Same as above.
22. Yang, W., et al. (2021). The association between maternal fat-soluble vitamin concentrations during pregnancy and infant birth weight in China. *British Journal of Nutrition,* 125(9):1058-1066.
23. "Vitamin A Deficiency and Infertility." (n.d.). IVF Phoenix. Retrieved from https://www.ivfphoenix.com/vitamin-a-deficiency-and-infertility/.
24. Clagett-Dame, M. & Knutson, D. (2011). Vitamin A in reproduction and development. *Nutrients,* 3(4):385-428.
25. Fung, J. L., et al. (2017). Association of vitamin D intake and serum levels with fertility: Results from the Lifestyle and Fertility Study. *Fertility & Sterility,* 108(2): 302–311.
26. Meng, X., et al. (2023). Influence of Vitamin D supplementation on reproductive outcomes of infertile patients: a systematic review and meta-analysis. *Reproductive Biology and Endocrinology,* 21: 17.
27. "Vitamin D" (n.d.). Root Cause Protocol. Retrieved from https://therootcauseprotocol.com/vit-d-faq/
28. Ware, Megan. (2023). "What are the benefits of cod liver oil?" Medical News Today. Retrieved from https://www.medicalnewstoday.com/articles/270071%23nutrition
29. Khan, Q. & Fabian, C. (2010). How I Treat Vitamin D Deficiency. *Journal of Oncology Practice,* 6(2): 97–101.
30. Institute of Medicine. (1998). Dietary Reference Intakes: Thiamin, Riboflavin, Niacin, Vitamin B6, Folate, Vitamin B12, Pantothenic Acid, Biotin, and Choline. Washington, DC: *National Academy Press.*
31. Zeisel, S. H. (2010). Choline. In P. M. Coates, J. M. Betz, M. R. Blackman, & et al. (Eds.), *Encyclopedia of Dietary Supplements* (2nd ed., pp. 136-143). London and New York: Informa Healthcare.

32. Zhan, X., et al. (2021). Choline supplementation influences ovarian follicular development. *Frontiers in Bioscience,* 26(12):1525-1536.
33. Same as above.
34. Korsmo, H., et al. (2019). Choline: Exploring the Growing Science on Its Benefits for Moms and Babies. *Nutrients,* 11(8): 1823.
35. Sanders, L. & Zeisel, S. (2007). Choline. *Nutrition Today,* 42(4): 181–186.
36. Zeisel, S. H., Mar, M. H., Zhou, Z. W., & da Costa, K. A. (1995). Pregnancy and lactation are associated with diminished concentrations of choline and its metabolites in rat liver. *Journal of Nutrition,* 125(12), 3049–3054.
37. Tonai, S., et al. (2022). Iron deficiency induces female infertile in order to failure of follicular development in mice. *The Journal of Reproduction and Development,* 66(5): 475–483.
38. Bermejo, F. & García-López, S. (2009). A guide to diagnosis of iron deficiency and iron deficiency anemia in digestive diseases. *World Journal of Gastroenterology,* 15(37): 4638–4643.
39. Ems, T., et al. (2023). Biochemistry, Iron Absorption. *StatPearls.* Treasure Island (FL): StatPearls Publishing.
40. Kamenju, P., et al. (2022). Higher Dietary Intake of Animal Protein Foods in Pregnancy Is Associated with Lower Risk of Adverse Birth Outcomes. *The Journal of Nutrition,* 152(11):2546-2554.
41. Mandal, U., et al. (2014). Management of experimental hypochlorhydria with iron deficiency by the composite extract of Fumaria vaillantii L. and Benincasa hispida T. in rat. *Journal of Natural Science, Biology, and Medicine,* 5(2): 397–403.
42. Lynch, S. R. & Cook, J. D. (1980). Interaction of vitamin C and iron. *Annals of the New York Academy of Sciences,* 355: 32-44.
43. Beck, K. & Coad, J. (2017). Dairy Product (Calcium) Consumption and Iron Nutrition. *Nutrients in Dairy and Their Implications on Health and Disease,* 149-160

44. Osazuwa, F., et al. (2011). A significant association between intestinal helminth infection and anaemia burden in children in rural communities of Edo state, Nigeria. *North American Journal of Medical Sciences,* 3(1): 30–34.
45. Jalambo, M., et al. (2018). Effects of iron supplementation and nutrition education on haemoglobin, ferritin and oxidative stress in iron-deficient female adolescents in Palestine: randomized control trial. *Eastern Mediterranean Health Journal,* 24(6).

Chapter 16: Dietary Strategies for Hormone Health

1. Weston A. Price Foundation. (2000). "Timeless Principles of Healthy Traditional Diets." *Wise Traditions.* Retrieved from https://www.westonaprice.org/health-topics/abcs-of-nutrition/principles-of-healthy-diets-2/#gsc.tab=0
2. Same as above.
3. Elango, R., & Ball, R. O. (2016). Protein and amino acid requirements during pregnancy. *Advances in Nutrition,* 7(4), 839S-844S.
4. "Fluid and Electrolyte Balance." (n.d.) *MedicinePlus.* Retrieved from https://medlineplus.gov/fluidandelectrolytebalance.html
5. Suba, Z. (2012). Interplay between insulin resistance and estrogen deficiency as co- activators in carcinogenesis. *Pathology and Oncology Research,* 18(2):123-33.
6. Haffner, S. M. (1996). Sex hormone-binding protein, hyperinsulinemia, insulin resistance and noninsulin-dependent diabetes. *Hormone Research,* 45(3-5):233-7.
7. Meczekalski, B., et al. (2014). Functional hypothalamic amenorrhea and its influence on women's health. *Journal of Endocrinological Investigation,* 37: 1049-1056.
8. Patrick, L. (2020). Diabetes and Toxicant Exposure. *Integrative Medicine: A Clinician's Journal,* 19(1): 16–23.
9. Mitrou, P., et al. (2015). Vinegar Consumption Increases Insulin-Stimulated Glucose Uptake by the Forearm Muscle in Humans with Type 2 Diabetes. *Journal of Diabetes Research,* 175204.

About the Author

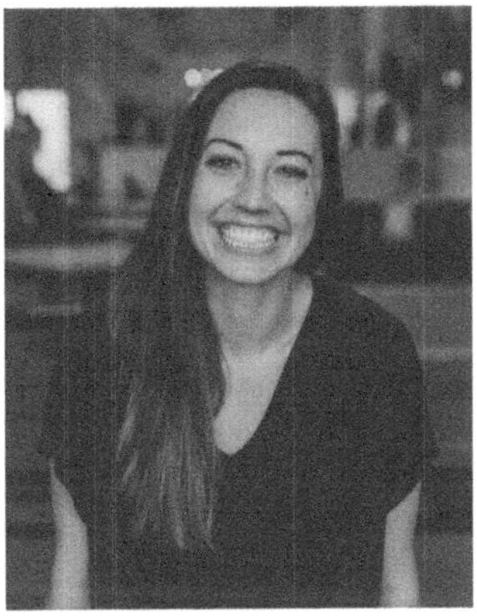

Deidre Bloomquist is a functional nutritionist and studying naturopathic doctor who owns Always Growing Nutrition, a virtual practice that serves clients across the United States. She leads a team of practitioners who work with women to resolve a wide range of digestive issues and hormone imbalances, as well as a dedicated pediatric practice. She specializes in reversing infertility by restoring health through reducing toxicity. She's an advocate of assessing toxin burden in the preconception phase to not only support fertility, but to promote he alth and healing for generations to come. She also teaches and mentors other practitioners to do this deep healing work with their clients.

To learn more, visit **www.always-growing.com.**

Made in United States
Cleveland, OH
24 October 2026

46774861R00181